The Language of Mental Health

This series brings together rich theoretical and empirical discussion at the intersection of mental health and discourse/conversation analysis. Situated broadly within a social constructionist perspective, the books included within this series will offer theoretical and empirical examples highlighting the discursive practices that surround mental health and make 'real' mental health constructs. Drawing upon a variety of discourse and conversation analysis perspectives, as well as data sources, the books will allow scholars and practitioners alike to better understand the role of language in the making of mental health.

Editorial Board

More information about this series at
http://www.palgrave.com/gp/series/15193

Joyce Lamerichs · Susan J. Danby · Amanda Bateman · Stuart Ekberg
Editors

Children and Mental Health Talk

Perspectives on Social Competence

palgrave
macmillan

Editors
Joyce Lamerichs
Department of Language, Literature and Communication
VU University Amsterdam
Amsterdam, Noord-Holland
The Netherlands

Amanda Bateman
Swansea University
Swansea, UK

Susan J. Danby
School of Early Childhood and Inclusive Education
Queensland University of Technology
Brisbane, QLD, Australia

Stuart Ekberg
School of Psychology and Counselling
Queensland University of Technology
Brisbane, QLD, Australia

The Language of Mental Health
ISBN 978-3-030-28425-1 ISBN 978-3-030-28426-8 (eBook)
https://doi.org/10.1007/978-3-030-28426-8

Cover illustration: Elena Ray/Alamy Stock Photo

This Palgrave Macmillan imprint is published by the registered company Springer Nature Switzerland AG
The registered company address is: Gewerbestrasse 11, 6330 Cham, Switzerland

Preface

This collection has arisen out of many years of shared research interests in exploring how children's social competence plays out in different institutional settings. We each have been involved in undertaking research in which a child's well-being and mental health constitute a focus of those investigations. Broadly within the contributions of this book, the authors present detailed analysis of naturally occurring social encounters based on interactions that involve children in a range of clinical, non-clinical and research settings. The focus of this book marks a watershed moment in that we attend to both the research component of understanding children's interactional competence in situ and also the role of the professional through their reflections.

This book grew out of seminars, activities and professional development programs for researchers and professionals to reflect together on research and professional insights. A seminar held at Queensland University of Technology in October 2016 titled 'Who is the expert here?' (led by Susan Danby and Stuart Ekberg) brought together researchers and professionals to share and reflect upon the research undertaken within a range of health and educational settings. The researchers discussed how their collaborations with the practitioners enriched the research practices, and the professionals considered what this might mean for their professional practices (e.g., see Houen, 2017). This approach optimises the usefulness of bringing together researchers and professionals to share their thinking in ways that produce more explanatory power than a single approach alone can do (McWilliam, 2012).

The power of these research-practice nexus conversations challenges existing ways where research may be privileged over practice. The conversations of professional reflections are consistent with the ongoing rise of 'applied conversation analysis' (Antaki, 2011). While Harvey Sacks' early work (1992) with the suicide prevention centre may be considered an example of applied conversation analysis, more recent initiatives more formally connect research with practice and, importantly, explicate the many lessons learned when working closely together with organisations (Kitzinger, 2011). There are complexities and difficulties, and possible discrepancies can exist between the language of professionals and the language of researchers using ethnomethodological and conversation analysis approaches (Peräkylä & Vehviläinen, 2003). For researchers, it is important to learn and engage with the language of professionals, to be able to communicate the findings from conversation analyses in ways that are recognisable and relevant to the organisation (Kitzinger, 2011).

Perhaps the most well-known method in the field of Conversation Analysis for using empirically based conversation analytic evidence to understand communication within organisations is the Conversation Analytic Role-play Method (CARM) (Stokoe, 2014). This approach uses audio and video recordings of actual encounters and then overlays these with a framework to discuss and understand how practitioners go about their mundane everyday work activities. This approach is a model of professional development that has produced new understandings to support practitioners and organisations to engage in effective communication practices. Building on CARM (Stokoe, 2014), others have brought together researchers and professionals with the aim to improve workplace communication. For instance, Church and Bateman have designed a method to engage in practical work with early childhood teachers (Church & Bateman, 2019). Known as the Conversation Analysis in Early Childhood (CAiEC) approach, the

CAiEC workshops (https://www.caiecworkshops.com) are philosophically structured within an interactional competence framework where teachers' professional knowledge is valued, and research and practice meet in collaborative and constructive ways to explore early childhood teaching strategies. As with CARM, CAiEC workshops use video footage of real-life practice as a discussion point with professionals around how particular practices support children's learning, stimulating reflection and informing both future practice and research. A similar focus on interactional strategies also is central to the Discursive Action Method (Lamerichs & te Molder, 2011), which has been used to invite adolescents and social workers to reflect on particular instances of their own talk and inspect the strategies they use. The method has since then been developed further and is currently used to guide different group of professionals to approach the communicative practices in which they engage as dialogical conversations (Aarts & Te Molder, 2017; see also https://www.centrumvoordialoog.nl).

What emerged from the interest in the researcher-professional connection is a series of chapters within this book that have the potential to reshape how we understand the nexus of research and professional practice. The aim of this book is to provide opportunities for complex conversations to emerge for researchers and professionals so that they can come together to genuinely access complex ways of thinking and doing around children's interactional competence. Our shared agenda formed a conceptual space where we realised that we needed to consider matters of the research and practice nexus within the current international policy and research environments to attend to the relevance of this work for organisations and to build sustainable relationships with stakeholders and organisations beyond academia. This broad range of professional reflections offers distinct perspectives of professional engagement with children. As such, their professional reflections bring a rich, holistic view of professional practices that take place in a range of settings addressed in this book.

The contributions of these chapters speak at a very practical level to global initiatives to orient to the contributions that research can make to fields outside of academia. Internationally, there is a new emphasis on the significant contributions that research practices can make to organisations outside academia. Researchers engaging with policy-makers, practitioners and professionals make possible the shared transfer of knowledge, methods and resources. For instance, the recently implemented national Australian Research Engagement and Impact Assessment was an initiative designed to reorient academic research agendas and practices to drive the work of businesses and to improve social and economic outcomes (Gunn & Mintrom, 2018). Within the New Zealand context, government initiatives such as the Teaching and Learning Research Initiative (TLRI) offer funding to support collaborative research between teachers and university researchers (http://www.tlri.org.nz). The TLRI incentive emphasises the importance of strong partnerships between teachers and researchers when applying for funding to ensure that teachers are recognised as professionals who competently identify areas of their professional practice that can be supported by research evidence. Within the Dutch context, the National Science Agenda 2019–2024 by the Ministry of Education, Culture and Science announced a focal area of research on children and youth (The Netherlands Initiative for Education Research (NRO), 2018). The research agenda identifies several subdomains (e.g., health care, education, psychosocial development and upbringing) in which transdisciplinary collaborations across professional organisations, scientists and policy-makers are proposed. These examples of policy initiatives are located within a national agenda.

Our intention as editors began with a different agenda. We set out to bring researcher-professional conversations closer to the everyday lives of researchers and professionals by focusing on local instances of engagement. Wishing to avoid the push and pull of national policy endeavours and associations with engagement and impact, we elected to situate this book within the foundational principles of ethnomethodology and conversation analysis by focusing on local practices and building capacity for re-shaping, at a very practical level, the kinds of relationships and interactions that can occur between researchers and professionals. What this means is that this book is intended to give genuine access to the complex ways that researchers and professionals can engage with each other, and to introduce potentially new converts to the power of rich conversations among researchers and professionals.

The overall goal of this undertaking is to embrace better opportunities to understand children and their interactional competence and, consequentially, children's contributions as key players in their everyday lives.

The Focus of This Book

The book examines the complex interplay of young children's interactional practices within a range of institutional settings. We take up the challenge of building a collection of documented research and professional practices and reflections. Each chapter first presents empirical research that investigates aspects of children's interactional practices, and this is followed by a section that is best described as a practice-led reflection. These chapters contribute to an emerging body of work that presents understandings of how children employ a range of interactional competences as they interact in clinical and other health settings with professionals whose role is to support the child's mental health and well-being. The chapters in this book take up the challenges of linking practice-led reflections by having invited professionals to reflect upon the research described in the first section of the chapter. Taken together, they provide rich accounts of the nexus of research and practice.

In *Children and Mental Health Talk: Perspectives on Social Competence*, the chapters are written by internationally known and respected researchers within the fields of studies of children through the lenses of ethnomethodology and conversation analysis, and many draw on the sociology of childhood and ethnomethodological understandings of social competence. An important feature of this book is that of professional reflections in response to the research reported in that chapter. This approach reflects the intention of the editors to bring to the fore the essential relationship that must exist for those who are researchers and those who are professionals within the field being researched.

This book consists of eight chapters that are book-ended by a first chapter that introduces the conceptual framing that underpins the book's philosophy and approach, and an epilogue (Chapter 8) that draws together the significance of this work. The remaining six chapters contribute to this book focus on 'the social arenas of action' (Hutchby & Moran-Ellis, 1998) of child-professional encounters, which we have categorised across three arenas of action: clinical encounters, non-clinical encounters and research encounters:

- Clinical encounters: *O'Reilly, Kiyimba and Hutchby* explore child mental health assessments conducted in the UK, highlighting the ways in which children display competence about their mental health in a clinical setting. *Kawashima and Maynard* consider echolalia by children diagnosed with autism spectrum disorder within a developmental disability clinic in the USA. By showing how children can use echolalia to accomplish particular social actions within clinical encounters, Kawashima and Maynard highlight some of the limitations of treating this phenomenon solely as a sign of mental health pathology.
- Non-clinical encounters: *Bateman and Danby* examine ways children discuss a potentially traumatic event in a non-clinical context. Focusing on discussions that occur within a New Zealand preschool about a recent earthquake, Bateman and Danby show how preschool teachers and children collaboratively contribute to discussions about their experiences of the earthquake, and routinely incorporated discussion of ways in which the local community was recovering from that experience. *Jol, Stommel and Spooren* explore Dutch police interrogations with children who have been the witness of a sexual offence, highlighting child interviewees' demonstrations of competence by reporting ways in which they misled offenders.
- Research encounters: *Theobald and Danby* consider mental well-being beyond a clinical context, by exploring a video-simulated research conversation in Australia. Through their analysis, Theobald and Danby highlight the children's competence when asked to discuss such potentially sensitive matters. *Lamerichs, Alisic and Schasfoort* consider displays of social competence in Dutch psychological research interviews about a traumatic event. Through their analysis of these encounters, Lamerichs and her colleagues show ways in which children skilfully resist attempts by the interviewing psychologist to pursue particular topical agendas.

Proposed as a series of researcher-professional conversations, the editors of this book aimed to bring to the fore the usefulness of conversations in terms of transdisciplinary knowledge translation.

Brisbane, Australia — Susan J. Danby
Brisbane, Australia — Stuart Ekberg
Swansea, UK — Amanda Bateman
Amsterdam, The Netherlands — Joyce Lamerichs

References

Aarts, N., & Te Molder, H. (2017). *Spreek, zwijg, lach, hoor, zie, vraag en verwonder… Een inleiding in de dialoog*. Wageningen, The Netherlands: Centrum voor Dialoog.

Antaki, C. (Ed.). (2011). *Applied conversation analysis: Intervention and change in institutional talk*. Basingstoke: Springer.

Church, A., & Bateman, A. (2019). Methodology and professional development: Conversation Analytic Role-play Method (CARM) for early childhood education. *Journal of Pragmatics, 143*, 242–254.

Gunn, A., & Mintrom, M. (2018). Measuring research impact in Australia *Australian Universities' Review, 60*(1), 9–15.

Houen, S. (2017). Teacher talk: "I wonder… request designs" (Thesis by publication). Queensland University of Technology, Brisbane, QLD, Australia. Retrieved from https://eprints.qut.edu.au/108029/1/Sandra_Houen_Thesis.pdf.

Hutchby, I., & Moran-Ellis, J. (1998). Situating children's social competence. In I. Hutchby & J. Moran-Ellis (Eds.), *Children and social competence: Arenas of action* (pp. 2–26). London: Falmer Press.

Kitzinger, C. (2011). Working with childbirth helplines: The contributions and limitations of conversation analysis. In C. Antaki (Ed.), *Applied Conversation Analysis* (pp. 98–118). London: Palgrave Macmillan.

Lamerichs, J., & te Molder, H. (2011). Reflecting on your own talk: The discursive action method at work. In C. Antaki (Ed.), *Applied conversation analysis: Intervention and change in institutional talk* (pp. 184–206). Houndsmills, Basingstoke, Hampshire: Palgrave Macmillan.

McWilliam, E. (2012). Foreword. In A. Lee & S. Danby (Eds.), *Reshaping doctoral education: International approaches and pedagogies* (pp. xvii–xxii). London: Routledge.

Peräkylä, A., & Vehviläinen, S. (2003). Conversation analysis and the professional stocks of interactional knowledge. *Discourse & Society, 14*(6), 727–750.

Stokoe, E. (2014). The Conversation Analytic Role-play Method (CARM): A method for training communication skills as an alternative to simulated role-play. *Research on Language and Social Interaction, 47*(3), 255–265.

The Netherlands Initiative for Education Research (NRO). (2018). *Knowledge agenda youth.* Retrieved from The Netherlands Initiative for Education Research (NRO), www.nro.nl/en/.

Acknowledgements

We would like to extend our gratitude to several people who have supported us during the development of this edited volume. We want to thank Michelle O'Reilly and Jessica Nina Lester, editors of the book series *The Language of Mental Health*, for considering this edited volume on Children and Mental health Talk as part of the series. We would also like to acknowledge Palgrave for supporting us throughout this process, particularly Joanna O'Neill for her help throughout.

This edited volume could not have been put together without the professionals, families and children who were involved in the studies included in this book. We thank all contributing authors for the time and energy they have put into writing up their work as well as all reviewers who helped us to improve and develop the chapters and the professional reflections prior to inclusion. Their participation has been vital and so has been the encouragement and support we received from of our partners, our families and our colleagues.

A Note on the Transcription System

In accordance with the standard approach taken in Conversation Analysis, the contributions to this volume report fragments of data that have been transcribed according to transcription conventions developed by Jefferson (2004), which record productional and distributional features of vocal conduct that have been found to be procedurally relevant to participants in interaction (Hepburn & Bolden, 2013). Sometimes, additional conventions developed by Mondada (2018) have been used to transcribe non-vocal embodied conduct. Readers who are not familiar with these conventions may wish to consult the following transcription key.

Temporal Dimensions

Wo[rd] [Wo]rd	Square brackets mark speaker overlap, with left square brackets indicating overlap onset and right square brackets indicating overlap offset.
Word=word	An equal sign indicates the absence of discernible silence between two utterances or actions, which can occur within a single person's turn or between the turns of two people.

Word (0.4) word	A number within parentheses refers to silence, which is measured to the nearest tenth of a second and can occur either as a pause within a current speaker's turn or as a gap between two speakers' turns.

Vocal Conduct

Word (.) word	A period within parentheses indicates a micropause of less than two-tenths of a second.
Word.	A period indicates falling intonation at the end of a unit of talk.
Word,	A comma indicates slightly rising intonation.
Word¿	An inverted question mark indicates moderately rising intonation.
Word;	Alternatively a semicolon also indicates moderately rising intonation.
Word?	A question mark indicates rising intonation.
Word_	An underscore following a word indicates level intonation.
Word	Underlining indicates emphasis being placed on the underlined sounds.
Wo:::rd	Colons indicate the stretching of the immediately preceding sound, with multiple colons representing prolonged stretching.
Wo::rd	Underlining followed by one or more colons indicates a shift in pitch during the pronunciation of a sound, with rising pitch on the underlined component followed by falling pitch on the colon component that is not underlined.
Wo::rd	An underlined colon indicates the converse of the above, with rising pitch on the underlined colon component.
↑Word↑	Upward arrows mark a sharp increased pitch shift, which begins in the syllable following the arrow. An utterance encased with upward arrows indicates that the talk is produced at a higher pitch than surrounding talk.

↓Word↓	Downward arrows mark a sharp decreased pitch shift, which begins in the syllable following the arrow. An utterance encased with downward arrows indicates that the talk is produced at a lower pitch than surrounding talk.
WORD	Upper case indicates talk produced at a louder volume than surrounding utterances by the same speaker.
°Word°	Words encased in degree signs indicate utterances produced at a lower volume than surrounding talk. Double degree signs indicate utterances produced at an every lower volume than surrounding talk.
>Word<	Words encased with greater-than followed by less-than symbols indicate talk produced at a faster pace than surrounding talk.
<Word>	Words encased with less-than followed by greater-than symbols indicate talk produced at a slower pace than surrounding talk.
Wor-	A hyphen indicates an abrupt termination in the pronunciation of the preceding sound.
£Word£	Pound signs encase utterances produced with smile voice.
#Word#	Hash signs encase utterances produced with creaky voice.
~Word~	Tilde signs encase utterances produced with tremulous voice.
hhh	The letter 'h' indicates audible exhalation, with more letters indicating longer exhalation.
.hhh	A period followed by the letter 'h' indicates audible inhalation.
→	Right arrows are used to highlight phenomena of interest.

((Description))	Words encased in double parentheses indicate aspects of conduct for which there is no established transcription convention. In many—but not all—chapters of this book, this convention is employed to transcribe embodied conduct. It is also used to convey issues that come up for researchers working with languages other than English. Alternatively, the below conventions are used to transcribe embodied conduct.

Embodied Conduct

% %	Percentage signs indicate the beginning and end of embodied actions of a particular participant.
* *	Asterisks are used to encase descriptions of embodied actions of another participant.
%--->	An arrow indicates an action continues across subsequent lines,
----->%	Until a corresponding arrow is reached.

References

Hepburn, A., & Bolden, G. B. (2013). The conversation analytic approach to transcription. In J. Sidnell & T. Stivers (Eds.), *The handbook of conversation analysis* (pp. 57–76). Chichester, West Sussex, UK: Wiley-Blackwell.

Jefferson, G. (2004). Glossary of transcript symbols with an introduction. In G. H. Lerner (Ed.), *Conversation analysis: Studies from the first generation* (pp. 13–31). Amsterdam: John Benjamins.

Mondada, L. (2018). Multiple temporalities of language and body in interaction: Challenges for transcribing multimodality. *Research on Language and Social Interaction, 51*(1), 85–106.

Contents

List of Professional Reflection Authors

Chapter 2 Nikki Kiyimba

Chapter 3 Tetsuya Abe

Chapter 4 Paula Robinson and Claire Lethaby

Chapter 5 Naomi Dessaur

Chapter 6 Gillian Busch

Chapter 7 Eva Alisic

Notes on Contributors

Tetsuya Abe is Associate Professor in the Department of Psychosomatic and General Internal Medicine at Kansai Medical University. Tetsuya Abe graduated from Osaka City University of Medicine in Japan and obtained his Doctor of Philosophy in Medicine at Kansai Medical University. For over 20 years, his practice has focused on functional gastrointestinal disorders and chronic non-malignant pain. He also works in the areas of conversation analysis, developmental disorders, medical interviews and medical education. He is a delegate of the Japanese Society of Psychosomatic Medicine.

Eva Alisic is Associate Professor, Child Trauma and Recovery, at the Melbourne School of Population and Global Health, University of Melbourne, Australia. She conducts research into how children and families cope with traumatic events such as disaster and violence, and works with policy makers and clinicians to translate research findings into practice.

Amanda Bateman began her career as an early childhood practitioner in Wales, UK, before completing her Ph.D. and moving to New Zealand to work as a Senior Lecturer in Early Childhood Education at

Waikato University. She is currently Senior Lecturer and Programme Director of Early Childhood Studies at Swansea University, Wales. In her research, Amanda Bateman uses ethnomethodology, conversation analysis and language socialisation theory to investigate the social worlds of children. She has been Principal Investigator for funded and non-funded research projects and is currently co-researcher on Royal Marsden and Teaching and Learning Research Initiative (TLRI) funded projects in New Zealand. Amanda Bateman has published widely from her research, including the books *Early Childhood Education: The Co-Production of Knowledge and Relationships*, and *Children's Knowledge-in-Interaction: Studies in Conversation Analysis.*

Gillian Busch is Senior Lecturer and Head of Program in early childhood at Central Queensland University (CQU), Rockhampton, Australia. Dr Busch uses ethnomethodology and conversation analysis to study interactions in family and education settings. She obtained her PhD from QUT with her thesis titled The Social Orders of Family Mealtime being awarded the Early Childhood Australia Doctoral Thesis Award in 2012. She is a co-editor of a book titled *Constructing Methodology for Qualitative Research: Researching Education and Social Practices*. She is involved in a number of research projects including family SKYPE interactions and celebrations in early childhood settings. Gillian is also an experienced early childhood teacher.

Jakob Cromdal is Professor of Educational Practice in the Department of Social and Welfare Studies, Linköping University, Sweden. He specialises in postcognitive approaches to social interaction which includes studies in ethnomethodology, conversation analysis, discursive psychology and membership categorisation analysis. He has published on a variety of topics related to young persons' social conduct within a variety of institutional settings such as classrooms, driving school cars, detention homes, emergency services and youth helplines.

Susan J. Danby is Professor in School of Early Childhood Education and Inclusive Education at Queensland University of Technology (QUT), Brisbane, Australia. Her research explores the everyday social and interactional practices of children, showing their complex and competent work as they build their social worlds with family members, peers and teachers within home and school contexts. She has published in the areas of qualitative research, helpline interaction, home and classroom interaction, early childhood pedagogy and doctoral education.

Naomi Dessaur is a Dutch social worker. She graduated from The Hague University of Applied Sciences and has a degree in advanced training as a coach, supervisor and trainer. After years of working with children and families, she saw how adults struggle to discuss subjects such as child abuse and sexuality with children. This 'invisible suffering' as she calls it was the trigger in 2008 to start with the Dessaur Training Company. She now trains professionals how to handle child abuse, domestic violence and sexual abuse and helps them to create a safe child-centred environment in which children can talk openly. She has also started an online platform to help parents/caregivers find ways to talk with children about sexuality and related issues.

Stuart Ekberg is a Senior Research Fellow in the School of Psychology & Counselling at Queensland University of Technology. He specialises in conversation analytic research, investigating social interaction across a range of settings. His current research focuses on psychotherapeutic interactions, paediatric palliative care consultations and mundane conversations. His work on this book was supported by a Discovery Early Career Researcher Award (Reference: DE170100026) from the Australian Research Council.

Ian Hutchby is an independent researcher, formerly Professor of Sociology at the University of Leicester, UK. His research uses conversation analysis to investigate the situated social competence of children interacting with adults in everyday and institutional settings such as child counselling, family therapy and child mental health assessments.

Guusje Jol is a Ph.D. candidate at the Centre for Language Studies at Radboud Universiteit Nijmegen, The Netherlands, and a Lecturer at the Open University. She has a background in both criminal law and linguistics. Her research interests include (institutional) interaction and language in a legal context.

Michie Kawashima is Associate Professor in the Department of International Studies at Kyoto Sangyo University in Japan. She has mainly worked on areas of conversation analysis and health communication. She has published widely on interpersonal interaction in women's health, palliative care, childcare and emergency medicine. Recent work has investigated how very bad news is delivered in a Japanese Emergency Room and interactional ('Mitori') practices in processes of death and dying at a Japanese Hospital.

Nikki Kiyimba is a Senior Educator and Programme Leader for the Masters in Professional Practice at Bethlehem Tertiary Institute, New Zealand. She also is a Chartered Clinical Psychologist, originally working in the UK specialising in working with clients experiencing complex trauma and enduring psychological difficulties, and now working with clients via Tele Health in New Zealand.

Joyce Lamerichs is Assistant Professor and an experienced researcher in the Faculty of Humanities at the Vrije Universiteit in Amsterdam, The Netherlands. Her research interests centre around institutional interactions in the domain of health. She has published in the areas of child and adult mental health, and combines insights from conversation analysis and discursive psychology to study both online and face-to-face encounters in health and medical settings. Her current research investigates end-of-life talk in Dutch University Medical Centres.

Claire Lethaby is the Assistant Centre Manager at New Brighton Community Preschool and Nursery. She has worked in this centre since 2002, as *kaiako* in both the preschool and infant and toddler areas. She is passionate about respectful practices and *tamariki* experiencing equality. Claire Lethaby has two sons, Quinn and Cullen, who have both joined her at the centre for their preschool years. In her spare time, she loves reading, crafting and crosswording as well as spending time with her family. Caravaning and camping is an important part of their family culture and they try to get away in their 1978 caravan called Jenny as much as possible, seeing the sights of beautiful Aotearoa.

Douglas W. Maynard is Conway-Bascom Professor, and Harold and Arlene Garfinkel Faculty Fellow in the Department of Sociology at the

University of Wisconsin–Madison. His current work includes co-editing (with John Heritage) a volume on Harold Garfinkel: Praxis, Social Order, and Ethnomethodology's Legacies (forthcoming with Oxford University Press), and a monograph co-authored with Jason Turowetz on the testing and diagnosis of Autism Spectrum Disorder (forthcoming with University of Chicago Press). At UW, he teaches undergraduate and graduate courses on ethnomethodology, on conversation analysis and on social psychology. He is the immediate past president of the International Society for Conversation Analysis.

Michelle O'Reilly is an Associate Professor of Communication in Mental Health at the University of Leicester, working for the Greenwood Institute of Child Health. Her joint activities between the university and Leicestershire Partnership NHS Trust centre on qualitative research in child mental health, with a focus on family therapy interactions and child mental health assessments.

Karin Osvaldsson Cromdal is a licensed psychologist with clinical experience from the Children and Youth Mental Health Services. She is Associate Professor of Child Studies in the Division of Social Work, Linköping University, Sweden. Osvaldsson Cromdal received her Ph.D. in Child Studies from Linköping University in 2002. Working within the main framework of ethnomethodology and discursive psychology, Osvaldsson is engaged in research on identity and social interaction in various settings, including detention homes for troubled youth, emergency rescue services and Internet and telephone counselling organisations. She is currently engaged in research projects on online social work counselling and child helpline organisations.

Paula Robinson is the Manager of New Brighton Community Preschool and Nursery and has been a member of this centre for over 20 years. Paula is passionate about this community and aims to make this centre a place where everyone feels this is their place. Paula's son Baxter attended the centre and now is at Intermediate School. He still loves coming into the centre now, acting as one of the team. Outside of work, Paula enjoys spending time cooking, doing crafts, watching Baxter's sports and having fun with her family. She loves the adventures that the countryside and weather offer, a sense her son also enjoys and her partner endures.

Marca Schasfoort is a University Teacher in the Department of Language, Literature and Communication at the Faculty of Humanities (Vrije Universiteit Amsterdam, The Netherlands). Marca Schasfoort has co-authored papers on institutional interaction and interactional analyses of psychological interviews with children who have experienced trauma. She teaches (applied) conversation analysis in the bachelor programme on communication and information studies. She is also an experienced trainer.

Wilbert Spooren is a Professor of Discourse Studies of Dutch (Centre for Language Studies, Radboud University Nijmegen, The Netherlands). His research interests are discourse and interaction analysis (with a particular focus on connectives and coherence relations in different genres), language use and effective communication, language use and new media, automatic analysis of coherence in text and talk, text structure and text quality and subjectivity in discourse.

Wyke Stommel is an Assistant Professor of Language and Communication in the Centre for Language Studies at Radboud University Nijmegen in The Netherlands. Her interests include interaction in institutional settings like counselling, the medical domain and the police.

Maryanne Theobald is Senior Lecturer in the School of Early Childhood and Inclusive Education at Queensland University of Technology (QUT), Brisbane, Australia. She has 20 years experience as an early childhood teacher. Her research focuses on communication practices and social interaction of children's participation, friendships, disputes, celebrations and peer cultures in classrooms, playgrounds, in multilingual and therapeutic settings. She has expertise in qualitative approaches including ethnomethodology and conversation analysis, and in transdisciplinary research with practitioner-researchers.

1

Professional Practices and Children's Social Competence in Mental Health Talk

Joyce Lamerichs, Stuart Ekberg, Amanda Bateman and Susan J. Danby

The World Health Organisation estimates that worldwide 10–20% of children and adolescents experience mental health problems (WHO, 2018). Beyond the boundaries of these clinically defined populations and conditions, children experience a range of ordinary and extraordinary circumstances that affect their mental health and wellbeing. Throughout their

J. Lamerichs (✉)
Department of Language, Literature and Communication, VU University Amsterdam, Amsterdam, Noord-Holland, The Netherlands
e-mail: j.m.w.j.lamerichs@vu.nl

S. Ekberg
School of Psychology and Counselling,
Queensland University of Technology, Brisbane, QLD, Australia
e-mail: stuart.ekberg@qut.edu.au

A. Bateman
Swansea University, Swansea, UK
e-mail: a.j.bateman@swansea.ac.uk

J. Lamerichs et al. (eds.), *Children and Mental Health Talk*,
The Language of Mental Health,
https://doi.org/10.1007/978-3-030-28426-8_1

lives, children may participate in a range of different institutional settings where emotional, behavioural and neurodevelopmental matters are attended to as relevant for the purposes of that institution. This might occur in clinical settings where mental health and wellbeing comprise a primary institutional focus. Beyond such institutions, the mental health and wellbeing of children also are of relevance in a range of other institutional settings, such as in educational or judicial systems or in the course of research. Studies in these different contexts show the differing understandings of children's interactions and a range of practices from those professionals who support children to manage their health and wellbeing. Rather than considering mental health and wellbeing issues as external forces that happen to the child, the perspective here taken is that children are directly involved in the process of talk around mental health issues in everyday contexts, positioning them as interactionally competent and capable. The undertaking of fine-grained analyses using ethnomethodological and conversation analysis approaches makes it possible to observe of the multifaceted ways that children manage and display social competence in a range of institutional settings.

From a Developmental to an Interactional Perspective on Children's Social Competence

The concept of children's competence often is framed as an assessment of children's capability. Claims of children as competent—or not—are driven by underlying paradigms that provide conceptual constructions of the child as developing competence, prominent in many sociological and psychological studies. As you read the chapters of this book, you will see that the theoretical framing of children's interactional competence is located and described as in situ competence. In this understanding,

S. J. Danby
School of Early Childhood and Inclusive Education,
Queensland University of Technology, Brisbane, QLD, Australia
e-mail: s.danby@qut.edu.au

first recognised by the early ethnomethodologists, we describe children as 'competent interpreters in the world' (Mackay, 1991: 31). The early ethnomethodologists, including Robert Mackay (1991) and Matthew Speier (1971, 1973), were the first to write about the social competence of children. Their pioneering work investigated children's interactional competence in everyday interactions, and this theoretical framing of children's competence can be located and described as in situ competences.

A sociological perspective recognises children as collaboratively producing and making sense of their worlds through their social interactions in everyday life and involves examining how children display their social competence in situ. For example, Danby and Baker (2000) showed how first impressions of young children's interactions can suggest that they have an undeveloped idea of turn taking, an essential feature of social interaction. A study of preschool-aged boys in the classroom showed how they talked over each other, so that they did not wait until one had finished their turn before another started. The talk gave the appearance of speaker turns being unorganised and jumbled. Yet detailed analysis showed that they were not engaging in interactions that were chaotic but, rather, the talk was ordered and systematic. The specific element for being heard was to have the speaker's main message audible; recycling their initial turns of talk that overlapped with another meant that their main message was heard in its entirety. The finding showed that young children's talk was not disorderly nor chaotic but that it used the same features as adult talk. As Schegloff (1987) found in adult conversations, adults routinely talk over each other to get the floor for speaking yet, as Danby and Baker (2000) found, 3- and 4-year-old children also do this to gain the floor. In our society, the developmental perspective is so persuasive that it is easy to think that the practice of children talking over each other is there because they have not learned to take turns at talk.

It is not always possible, though, for children to engage in the conversations that are about them or involve them in some way. Children often are not afforded the opportunity to be included and, even when they are included, they elect to not contribute to the talk about them or involving them, even when asked. One way in which children can display their competence is by resisting engagement in discussions about their mental health (Hutchby, 2002; O'Reilly & Parker, 2013). One well-documented practice that children use is to disclaim knowledge with expression such as 'I don't know' (Hutchby, 2002; Lamerichs, Alisic, & Schasfoort, 2018; O'Reilly, Lester, & Muskett, 2016; Stafford, Hutchby, Karim, & O'Reilly, 2016; Stickle, Duck, & Maynard, 2017). There is no reason, however, to assume that these knowledge disclaimers index a state of mental incompetence. For example, Hutchby (2002) considers an example from a child counselling session where a child client responds with 'don't know' to 57 of the 92 questions asked by his counsellor. The following fragment shows two of these responses:

Fragment 1 (Hutchby, 2002: 160)

```
((Referring to the child's drawing))
01     C:  Is that da:d. in Paris,
02         (2.1)
03     C:  Who's this in Paris,
04 → P:  °Don't know,°
05     C:  No who is it, an-=seriously who is it.
06 → P:  °Don't know.°
07         (.)
08     C:  Jus' people,
09         (1.6)
10     C:  °Mm.°
```

The child first disclaims knowledge at line 4. Given that what is being disclaimed is knowledge about a picture that he has just drawn, this response is treated as non-serious by the counsellor, rather than an indication of the child's actual mental state. Here and elsewhere in this session, disclaiming knowledge is employed by the child client to continue avoiding the counsellor's questions, even after his pursuit of a serious response. Disclaiming knowledge highlights the socially competent ways that children resist engaging in encounters that they may be involved in against their own volition (Hutchby, 2002).

Ethnomethodological and Conversation Analysis Approaches for Understanding Mental Health Talk with Children

Ethnomethodological and conversation analysis approaches to analysing child mental health talk make possible fine-grained analysis that displays evidence of how children engage in these conversations. First, children can find themselves often engaging with mental health professionals due to decisions that have been made by adults rather than by themselves (Fasulo, 2015; Hutchby, 2002; O'Reilly & Parker, 2013; Stafford et al., 2016). Indeed, in some situations a child's conduct may even suggest that they are unclear about why a decision has been made to bring them to such a setting (Kiyimba, O'Reilly, & Lester, 2018). Second, in some settings, such as family therapy, the presence of other parties, such as family members, can affect the extent and way in which children participate in mental health talk (Hutchby & O'Reilly, 2010; O'Reilly & Parker, 2014). Third, children may be treated in ways that position them as more or less knowledgeable about their own mental health and wellbeing (Butler, Potter, Danby, Emmison, & Hepburn, 2010; O'Reilly et al., 2016).

Professionals who engage children in mental health talk seek to find ways of broaching this potentially delicate matter in ways that suit individual children and their circumstances. Recent years have seen a rapid increase in research exploring practices that professionals can use to pursue this objective. Although this body of research remains relatively small, it nonetheless already contributes a range of practical guidance. At a general level, the findings of this research identify a broad spectrum of practices that professionals use to promote mental health talk. Practices towards one end of this spectrum attempt to bring into direct focus matters that are relevant to a child's mental health and wellbeing, while practices towards the opposite end of this spectrum are used to discuss a child's mental health and wellbeing more indirectly. We consider practices towards either end of this spectrum in turn.

There are circumstances where it is ostensibly relevant for a professional to take, as a direct focus, a child's mental wellbeing. For example, one practical task for child counsellors to focus on matters that are relevant for counselling. This can be seen in the following fragment, where the counsellor (C) comes to directly and explicitly highlight the emotional impact of the child client's (referred to as J) circumstances:

Fragment 2 (Hutchby, 2005: 317–318)

```
01 C:  A::h 'kay so if you did what your da:d (.)
02     a::sked you or suggested, li[ke ] go an' play on the=
03 J:                             [Yeh]
04 C:  =computer, (0.5) would that happen would your mum an' dad
05     have an argument about it.
06 J:  Well they- the:y wouldn't me an' my mum would an' me an'
07     my dad would. .hh An' my mum an' dad would tell each
08     other off but they wouldn't argue.
09 C:  A::h. (.) Is that, different do [they
10 J:                                  [An' my mum would smack
11     me an' send me up t' bed. [Even-
   ((22 lines omitted))
33 C:  D'you think she'd prefer to smack dad.
34     (.)
35 J:  No:.
36     (0.8)
37 J:  Cuz dad would smack her back an' then, .h they'd have a
38     big fight on smacking.
39 C:  A big smacking fight.
40 J:  Yeah.=
41 C:  =That doesn't sound like a ver[y nice (thing)
42 J:                                [No: so I just take the
43     smack an' I don't really care (cuz) she can't- .hh well
44     she can smack really hard but it doesn't hu:rt.
45 C:  So::, so 'f she smacks you::, (.) sometimes it might feel
46     better cuz it means that mum and dad don't have a row.
47 J:  Yeh.
48 C:  A:::h. 'Ka::y.
```

In this fragment, the child client describes a circumstance in which she can come to be smacked by her mother. After some discussion of this matter (not all of which is reported here), the counsellor formulates an upshot of the discussion that focuses on the emotional impact of this circumstance upon the client (lines 45–46). This brings into direct focus an aspect of the client's mental wellbeing—her emotions—that has not been made explicit in the prior talk. Other research identifies alternative practices that therapists use to ground mental health talk in something that has already been raised by the child client (Danby & Emmison, 2014; Kiyimba & O'Reilly, 2018; O'Reilly, Kiyimba, & Karim, 2016). What is common across these practices they make discussion of mental health or wellbeing direct and explicit.

On the other hand, there are also practices that professionals use to focus on mental health and wellbeing more indirectly. For example, fictional characters (Lester & O'Reilly, 2015) and metaphors (Bradley & Butler, 2015) can work to create a social distance between a child's behaviour and their broader identity, so the child can critically discuss their behaviour without associating this with their identity more broadly. For instance, in the fragment below we see an example of how reference to the superhero character *Superflex*, who was considered capable to defeat a range of social and behavioural problems, referred to as 'unthinkables'. As we see in the fragment, 'Glassman' is used as a reference to one of the 'unthinkables' (line 4), corresponding to a situation in which the child would make a small problem into a big problem that resulted in what was called an 'earth shattering reaction' (Lester & O'Reilly, 2015: 340). These references to unthinkables and the superhero enabled the therapist to address and negotiate the boundaries of what are inappropriate and appropriate behaviours. At the same time, they position the child as capable of dealing with inappropriate behaviour. In Fragment 3, Bria is the therapist and Billy is the child.

Fragment 3 (Lester & O'Reilly, 2015: 340)

```
01 Bria:   First you pick and then I get to pick (2) kay=
02 Billy:  (Climbs on to the swing) (3)
03 Bria:   (Pushes swing) thank you for being Superflex and using a
04         nice voice (1) for a second there I thought Glassman was
05         gonna come [out
06 Billy:             [Whoa (.)
07 Bria:   You were almost being kind of rude but [then↑
08 Billy:                                         [ah (.)
09 Bria:   out comes Superflex↑
```

In instances where initial attempts to elicit mental health talk falter, there are alternative strategies that professional child counsellors and therapists can use to more indirectly foster talk on delicate matters. For example, professionals have successfully promoted discussion by asking children to engage in drawing activities that allow them to communicate about a sensitive matter in a different way (Fogarty, Augoustinos, & Kettler, 2013). Nevertheless, as illustrated in Fragment 1 above, drawing activities do not guarantee success in promoting sensitive conversations (Hutchby, 2002). No single practice is guaranteed to be successful but, rather, professionals who interact with children draw on a repertoire of practices that are suitable for a particular child and their immediate circumstances.

There is a broader range of professionals—not only those working within clinical settings—who may find themselves in circumstances where they engage with children about matters that relate to their mental health and wellbeing. For instance, educators often are afforded opportunities to engage in particular types of encounters that incorporate discussions of mental wellbeing that may not be possible in mental health settings. For example, early childhood teachers and children can embed discussions of traumatic events within activities that routinely occur as part of early childhood education (Bateman & Danby, 2013). One effective device used by the early childhood teachers in a study around post-earthquake play in New Zealand was that of second stories, where the teacher encouraged children to produce second stories on hearing a first story about the earthquake event. In this way, talk became an interactional resource to shift accounts from the earthquake itself to the relational aspects of community support (Bateman & Danby, 2013). Nevertheless, as in the mental health settings considered earlier, children may not align with attempts to initiate such talk (Bateman, Danby, & Howard, 2013). In the following fragment (considered in detail in Chapter 4), and in contrast to the prior child counsellor fragments, here it is the child who initiates talk about his earthquake experience. In the mundane context of sitting on the grass reading books, the child (ZAC) selects a story he had written about his earthquake experience directly after the event and gives it to his teacher (LEO) to read to him:

Fragment 4 (Bateman & Danby, 2013)

```
ZAC:   ↑now can you read ↓mi:ne:?
LEO:   ar=↑sure:↓ . and that was all about the ↓earthquake
       wasn't it >remember=when=we< had the
       <earthqu:ake::> can you remember about the
       earth↑quake::?
ZAC:   ↑yeah↑=
LEO:   =what can you remember about the earth↑quake¿
ZAC:   [ ↑ m m m m ¿ ]              [we:: (        )]
LEO:   [wha:t special] thing could [↑you remember¿]
ZAC:   on the grass?
LEO:   we did did↑n't we::¿ . and we all [came on to-]
ZAC:                                     [↑I remember] we-
       I remember- I remember it?
LEO:   ↑you rem↓ember it? ↓can you remember what happened?
       (0.9)
ZAC:   °mmm the dinosaurs-° the ↑di:nosaurs were dancing¿
LEO:   the ↑dinosaurs were dancing¿
       (0.7)
LEO:   ↑real:ly:¿
```

Although this educational context is different to clinical settings, the professional practice of eliciting talk about a traumatic event from a child is still evident. What is clear is that professionals who seek to engage children in mental health talk approach this delicate matter in ways that align with children's immediate contexts. The approach taken by the professional reflects the specific professional context in which the talk is embedded.

There is a range of ways in which professional contexts can influence mental health talk with children. Some contexts involve regulation about what professionals can and cannot do. For example, Kids Helpline is an Australian helpline for children and young people, where counsellors respond to young callers and provide counselling support through telephone, online chat and email modalities. They draw on strategies that include designing the opening of the calls for callers to find their own way into their reason for calling the helpline (Danby, Baker, & Emmison, 2005) working within the institutional remit of 'We listen, we care'. In enacting this remit, the counsellors avoided giving advice, even when requested by the caller (Butler et al., 2010). Rather, they used strategic questions to afford agency to the caller to solve their own problems, and other strategies that included using address terms to build client rapport and trust (Butler, Danby, & Emmison, 2011), script proposals to propose what a caller might say to a third party (Emmison, Butler, & Danby, 2011), compliment-giving to help callers identify their strengths (Danby, Butler, & Emmison, 2011), respecification of the clients' troubles (Cromdal, Danby, Emmison, Osvaldsson, & Cobb-Moore, 2018) and counsellor displays of active listening (Danby, Butler, & Emmison, 2009). Acknowledging children's competencies in mental health talk is imperative in ensuring that the wellbeing of the child is supported in such a sensitive context.

Beyond the specific practices that professionals use to facilitate discussions about mental health and wellbeing, establishing and maintaining good rapport with a child is an important foundation for promoting discussions about these matters. Although establishing rapport at the outset of an encounter is important (Childs & Walsh, 2017), rapport is to be actively maintained over time, especially during periods of sensitive and challenging discussions (Fogarty et al., 2013; Iversen, 2019). In multiparty settings such as family therapy, professionals must find ways to simultaneously maintain rapport with parties who are likely to hold divergent perspectives (Parker & O'Reilly, 2012). As professionals attempt to promote and sustain talk about a child's mental health and wellbeing, they work towards establishing and maintaining a relationship to facilitate such conversation.

Recent years have seen a rapid increase in exploring practices in different professional settings that pursue specific objectives. The practices range from specific practices that professionals use to directly or indirectly engage children in mental health talk, through to practices that more generally facilitate a productive relationship that appears necessary for such conversations to occur. Although this body of research remains relatively small and is restricted to only a small number of institutional contexts where mental health and wellbeing talk occurs, it nonetheless highlights a range of practices that professionals use to foster conversations about mental health and wellbeing with children.

Professional Practices and Professional Vision

Professionals at work provide the backdrop to the concept of professional vision, which underpins the work discussed in the chapters of this book. This concept was coined by Charles Goodwin (1994) and is defined as 'socially organized ways of seeing and understanding events that are answerable to the distinctive interests of a particular social group' (Goodwin, 1994: 606). This concept is one way to understand how professional groups orient to how they go about producing their professional knowledge in ways that other professionals recognise as institutional work. Professionals orient to specific features of the physical and social environment. Goodwin initially demonstrated this concept through analysis of video footage of archaeologists going about their everyday work, and then he elaborated his concept through the analysis of police officers in courtroom encounters. In both these examples, Goodwin's point was that professionals attended to some certain features of the environment, and not to others, focusing on what is important to the participants as professionals in that place and that time.

Goodwin (1994) suggests that people working in the same profession (e.g. child counsellors) speak a common language and enact being a professional as expected by other members of the profession. In this way, professional vision is interactively organised and situated as orienting to specific aspects relevant to the profession is observable within a specific profession. Not only do professionals organise their work through their own conduct, they also make noticings of others' conduct to co-produce situated practice, bringing some features into focus while not attending to others. Hutchby (2015: 541) has translated this vision to the setting of child counselling, for the purpose of which he has coined the term 'therapeutic vision' to refer broadly to 'seeing and understanding events according to occupationally relevant norms' (p. 149). For example, child counsellors routinely highlight aspects of a child's talk that can be considered relevant for addressing matters relevant to the child's feelings. Hutchby sees those 'counselling-relevant frames' laid down in the context of manuals or storybooks. This professional attention constitutes the production of an institutional approach to professional practice.

The concept of professionals having a vision to notice things relevant to their work in settings in which child mental health becomes a focus is mirrored by Peräkylä and Vehviläinen (2003). They introduced the notion of professional 'stocks of interactional knowledge' (SIKs) to refer to the 'normative models and theories or quasi-theories about interaction' that professionals draw on in their work and when they talk about what it is they do (2003: 729–730). These normative models are deeply constitutive of the relevant institutional practices that professionals rely on in their professional orientation to work practices. Peräkylä and Vehviläinen use psychotherapy as an example of an institutional setting in which the SIK that underly psychotherapy is highly constitutive of the praxis, or as the authors claim, without SIKs, there would be no psychotherapy.

A primary contribution by Peräkylä and Vehvilainen's (2003) is the articulation of how findings drawn from ethnomethodological and conversation analysis relate to professionals' theories about their interactional practices. In so doing, they identified particular directions in which these studies contribute to exemplifying SIKs that may only be described in very general terms and thus help to further explicate the professional theories and normative principles that operate in these domains. For example, Danby, Emmison, and Butler (2009) and Hutchby (2005) explored the therapeutic concept of 'active listening', highlighting the ways in which it is accomplished 'as part of the practical, contingent, and interactionally skilful work of counsellors and children as cultural members, rather than the abstract recommendations of handbooks and training manuals' (Hutchby, 2005: 309). Brought to the fore are profession-relevant concepts and strategies oriented to by the professionals in the course of their everyday work practices.

Professionals work in specific ways that are framed by their stocks of interactional knowledge (SIKs) and their professional vision to do what is required of them in their everyday work. In this sense, professional vision is observable as a universal phenomenon that frames each professionals' practice. Nevertheless, each professional's vision is enacted differently within the confines of the specific professional contexts. The chapters within this book highlight a diverse range of interactional practices that professionals use to facilitate talk with children about mental health and wellbeing.

In doing so, these chapters consider ways in which professional practices interface with children's competence.

References

Bateman, A., & Danby, S. (2013). Recovering from the earthquake: Early childhood teachers and children collaboratively telling stories about their experiences. *Disaster Prevention and Management, 22*(5), 467–479.

Bateman, A., Danby, S., & Howard, J. (2013). Living in a broken world: How young children's well-being is supported through playing out their earthquake experiences. *International Journal of Play, 2*(3), 202–219.

Bradley, L., & Butler, C. W. (2015). Managing and normalising emotions in behaviour: A conversation analytic study of ADHD coaching. In M. O'Reilly & J. N. Lester (Eds.), *The Palgrave handbook of child mental health* (pp. 480–499). Basingstoke: Palgrave Macmillan.

Butler, C. W., Danby, S., & Emmison, M. (2011). Address terms in turn beginnings: Managing disalignment and disaffiliation in telephone counselling. *Research on Language & Social Interaction, 44*(4), 338–358.

Butler, C. W., Potter, J., Danby, S., Emmison, M., & Hepburn, A. (2010). Advice-implicative interrogatives: Building "client-centered" support in a children's helpline. *Social Psychology Quarterly, 73*(3), 265–287.

Childs, C., & Walsh, D. (2017). Self-disclosure and self-deprecating self-reference: Conversational practices of personalization in police interviews with children reporting alleged sexual offenses. *Journal of Pragmatics, 121,* 188–201.

Cromdal, J., Danby, S., Emmison, M., Osvaldsson, K., & Cobb-Moore, C. (2018). "Basically it's the usual whole teen girl thing": Stage-of-life categories on a children and young people's helpline. *Symbolic Interaction, 41*(1), 25–44.

Danby, S., & Baker, C. (2000). Unravelling the fabric of social order in block area. In S. Hester & D. Francis (Eds.), *Local educational order: Ethnomethodological studies of knowledge in action* (pp. 91–140). Amsterdam: John Benjamins.

Danby, S., Baker, C., & Emmison, M. (2005). Four observations on opening calls to Kids Help Line. In C. Baker, M. Emmison, & A. Firth (Eds.), *Calling for help: Language and social interaction in telephone helplines* (pp. 133–151). Amsterdam and Philadelphia: John Benjamins.

Danby, S., Butler, C. W., & Emmison, M. (2009). When 'listeners can't talk': Comparing active listening in opening sequences of telephone and online counselling. *Australian Journal of Communication, 36*(3), 91–114.
Danby, S., Butler, C. W., & Emmison, M. (2011). 'Have you talked with a teacher yet?': How helpline counsellors support young callers being bullied at school. *Children and Society, 25*(4), 328–339.
Danby, S., & Emmison, M. (2014). Kids, counselors and troubles-telling: Morality-in-action in talk on an Australian children's helpline. *Journal of Applied Linguistics and Professional Practice, 9*(2), 99–120.
Emmison, M., Butler, C. W., & Danby, S. (2011). Script proposals: A device for empowering clients in counselling. *Discourse Studies, 13*(1), 3–26.
Fasulo, A. (2015). The value of conversation analysis for the study of children's mental health. In M. O'Reilly & J. N. Lester (Eds.), *The Palgrave handbook of child mental health* (pp. 3–24). Basingstoke: Palgrave Macmillan.
Fogarty, K., Augoustinos, M., & Kettler, L. (2013). Re-thinking rapport through the lens of progressivity in investigative interviews into child sexual abuse. *Discourse Studies, 15*(4), 395–420.
Goodwin, C. (1994). Professional vision. *American Anthropologist, 96*(3), 606–633.
Hutchby, I. (2002). Resisting the incitement to talk in child counselling: Aspects of the utterance 'I don't know'. *Discourse Studies, 4*(2), 147–168.
Hutchby, I. (2005). "Active listening": Formulations and the elicitation of feelings-talk in child counselling. *Research on Language and Social Interaction, 38*(3), 303–329.
Hutchby, I. (2015). Therapeutic vision: Eliciting talk about feelings in child counselling for family separation. In M. O'Reilly & J. N. Lester (Eds.), *The palgrave handbook of child mental health*. Houndmills, Basingstoke, UK: Palgrave Macmillan.
Hutchby, I., & O'Reilly, M. (2010). Children's participation and the familial moral order in family therapy. *Discourse Studies, 12*(1), 49–64.
Iversen, C. (2019). Beyond accessing information: Claiming to understand in child social welfare interviews. *British Journal of Social Psychology, 58*(3), 550–568.
Kiyimba, N., & O'Reilly, M. (2018). Reflecting on what 'you said' as a way of reintroducing difficult topics in child mental health assessments. *Child and Adolescent Mental Health, 23*(3), 148–154.
Kiyimba, N., O'Reilly, M., & Lester, J. N. (2018). Agenda setting with children using the 'three wishes' technique. *Journal of Child Health Care, 22*(3), 419–432.

Lamerichs, J., Alisic, E., & Schasfoort, M. (2018). Accounts and their epistemic implications: An investigation of how 'I don't know' answers by children are received in trauma recovery talk. *Research on Children and Social Interaction, 2*(1), 25–48.

Lester, J. N., & O'Reilly, M. (2015). The discursive construction of problem behaviours of children with autism in therapy. In M. O'Reilly & J. N. Lester (Eds.), *The Palgrave handbook of child mental health* (pp. 332–349). Basingstoke: Palgrave Macmillan.

Mackay, R. W. (1991). Conceptions of children and models of socialization. In F. C. Waksler (Ed.), *Studying the social worlds of children: Sociological readings* (pp. 23–37). London: Falmer Press.

O'Reilly, M., Kiyimba, N., & Karim, K. (2016a). "This is a question we have to ask everyone": Asking young people about self-harm and suicide. *Psychiatric and Mental Health Nursing, 23*(8), 479–488.

O'Reilly, M., Lester, J. N., & Muskett, T. (2016b). Children's claims to knowledge regarding their mental health experiences and practitioner's negotiation of the problem. *Patient Education and Counseling, 99*(6), 905–910.

O'Reilly, M., & Parker, N. (2013). You can take a horse to water but you can't make it drink': Exploring children's engagement and resistance in family therapy. *Contemporary Family Therapy, 35*(3), 491–507.

O'Reilly, M., & Parker, N. (2014). 'She needs a smack in the gob': Negotiating what is appropriate talk in front of children in family therapy. *Journal of Family Therapy, 36*(3), 287–307.

Parker, N., & O'Reilly, M. (2012). 'Gossiping' as a social action in family therapy: The pseudo-absence and pseudo-presence of children. *Discourse Studies, 14*(4), 457–475.

Peräkylä, A., & Vehviläinen, S. (2003). Conversation analysis and the professional stocks of interactional knowledge. *Discourse & Society, 14*(6), 727–750.

Schegloff, E. A. (1987). Recycled turn beginnings: A precise repair mechanism in conversation's turn-taking organisation. In G. Button & J. R. E. Lee (Eds.), *Talk and social organisation.* Clevedon: Multilingual Matters Ltd.

Speier, M. (1971). The everyday world of the child. In J. D. Douglas (Ed.), *Understanding everyday life* (pp. 188–217). London: Routledge.

Speier, M. (1973). *How to observe face-to-face communication: A sociological introduction.* Pacific Palisades, CA: Goodyear Publishing Company.

Stafford, V., Hutchby, I., Karim, K., & O'Reilly, M. (2016). "Why are you here?" Seeking children's accounts of their presentation to Child and Adolescent Mental Health Service (CAMHS). *Clinical Child Psychology and Psychiatry, 21*(1), 3–18.

Stickle, T., Duck, W., & Maynard, D. W. (2017). Children's use of "I don't know" during clinical evaluations for autism spectrum disorder: Responses to emotion questions. In M. O'Reilly, J. N. Lester, & T. Muskett (Eds.), *A practical guide to social interaction research in autism spectrum disorders* (pp. 247–273). London: Palgrave Macmillan.
World Health Statistics. (2018). *Monitoring health for the SDGs: Sustainable development goals.* Geneva: World Health Organization. Licence: CC BY-NC-SA 3.0 IGO.

2

Testing Children's Degrees and Domains of Social Competence in Child Mental Health Assessments

Michelle O'Reilly, Nikki Kiyimba and Ian Hutchby

Professional Reflection by Nikki Kiyimba

Introduction

In the UK, when there are concerns about a child's mental health, General Practitioners (GPs) make referrals to community mental health teams for specialist psychiatric assessments. The focus for this chapter is on exploring social competence of children within these initial child mental health assessments. The data analysed were video-recorded clinical conversations

M. O'Reilly (✉) · I. Hutchby
University of Leicester, Leicester, UK
e-mail: mjo14@leicester.ac.uk

N. Kiyimba
Bethlehem Tertiary Institute, Tauranga, New Zealand
e-mail: n.kiyimba@bti.ac.nz

J. Lamerichs et al. (eds.), *Children and Mental Health Talk*,
The Language of Mental Health,
https://doi.org/10.1007/978-3-030-28426-8_2

between mental health practitioners, children, young people and their families. We utilised conversation analysis (CA) to interrogate sequences of talk and investigate displays of category-bound developmental expectations. The analysis demonstrated how practitioners oriented to children's epistemic rights to knowing about their own mental state and motives for their behaviour. However, in terms of interactional competence, practitioners treated them as having degrees of competence in relation to understanding and appropriately articulating their mental state. When children and young people presented candidate diagnoses, such as 'self-harm', 'phobia' and 'OCD', practitioners did not overtly challenge their competence to understand these medical concepts, but did pursue further elaboration and ultimately confirmed or disconfirmed their proposition. The implications and applications of the analysis are therefore discussed later in the chapter.

The Literature

Conversation analysis (CA) has adopted a certain perspective on the question of children's participation both in everyday social life and in the institutional contexts that promote facilitation and mediation between adults and children. Broadly speaking, CA addresses children's talk in much the same way as it addresses adults' talk; that is, in terms of how it evidences the competent management of resources-at-hand to engage in social interaction that is meaningful, and displayed as such, for the participants in their local (social, temporal, interpersonal) circumstances (Hutchby & Wooffitt, 2008; Sacks, 1995). CA thus has affinities with the 'competence paradigm' in the sociology of childhood (James & Prout, 1990; Hutchby & Moran-Ellis, 1998).

In the competence paradigm, the question of children's social competence has often been contrasted with the focus on cognitive and social development that tends to characterise research in child psychology. A key argument has been that rather than being treated merely as bearers of developmental mechanisms, children need to be seen as social agents and active participants in their own social worlds. Indeed, sociological perspectives of childhood have challenged the views of children *developing* competence (see, e.g., Mackay, 1991; Prout & James, 1997), as this encourages a view of children as 'incomplete versions of adults' (Danby, 2002: 25). A resulting picture, therefore, emerges of childhood and adolescence as a 'dynamic arena of social activity involving struggles for power, contested meanings and negotiated relationships, rather than the linear picture of development and maturation made popular by traditional sociology and developmental psychology' (Hutchby & Moran-Ellis, 1998: 9). Thus, the competencies of children can be considered an interactional achievement in situ, within the local social setting, as opposed to an adult imposed assessment of capability (Theobald, 2016). For example, in relation to language competence it can be shown that children, even as young as 3–4 years old have a grasp of communication rules (Danby, 2002).

In many areas of their everyday lives, children and young people find themselves managing the contingencies of adult-controlled institutions, including not just the family home, but also school classrooms (Danby & Baker, 1998; Mayall, 1994), medical settings (Silverman, 1987; Stivers, 2002), and occasionally, for some, services such as counselling and mediation (Hutchby, 2007; Hutchby & O'Reilly, 2010). These settings involve practitioners and other organisational representatives who engage in task-oriented interaction with children and young people. One key theme often drawn out in relation to such settings is the way that differing epistemic perspectives can inform the participation of adults and children. Institutional forms of talk bring into play distinctive factors associated with the specific activities oriented to as relevant by different actors in the setting.

There is a twofold relevance to studying these differences. First, they can reveal how children and young people exercise their situated social competencies in orienting to those institutional agendas. Second, they can illuminate the ways in which practitioners, other professionals and policymakers themselves understand (or fail to understand) the social competencies of children and young people.

The Project

Children's competence is navigated, negotiated and displayed in a variety of mundane and institutional settings. In institutional environments, where children and young people are central to the institutional task, the importance of accurately determining competence has greater consequences as generally there is more at stake. One setting where the child's cognitive, social and emotional competence is frequently highlighted is during mental health assessments whereby mental health status relies heavily on self-report and family narratives about their thoughts, feelings and intentions. In that sense, competence is intrinsically bound to this in that clinical practitioners are faced with the task of deciphering whether the child or young person has sufficient competence to accurately report on matters that affect them. Thus, clinical practitioners tend to question and verify children's responses against adult versions to establish their accuracy in relation to the institutional task.

Context and Setting

Typically, in the UK, when families (or educators) have concerns about a child's mental health, parents usually attend an appointment with a General Practitioner (GP) to discuss their needs. The GP is thus usually the first point of contact for mental health problems and serves a gatekeeping function to making decisions regarding whether a referral to specialist services might be required or whether the problem can be managed in primary care. If a GP feels that the child or young person may have needs that warrant specialist mental health intervention, he or she will make a referral to the local Child and Adolescent Mental Health Service (CAMHS) requesting an initial assessment (Karim, 2015). In cases where there is enough information in the referral and grounds to do so, CAMHS will invite the family to attend an assessment appointment.

This assessment has many functions, including the assessment of symptoms and behaviours, evaluation of social circumstances and risk assessment (Sands, 2004). Practitioners also seek to ascertain some context about the child or young person's life (Mash & Hunsley, 2005), and this environment requires a great many questions to be asked of the family (O'Reilly, Karim, & Kiyimba, 2015). The questioning generally follows a similar pattern. Initial assessments tend to follow the trajectory of introductions, establishing reasons for attendance, ascertaining the nature of the problem (which includes establishing risk), reaching a decision and closing the session (O'Reilly, Karim, Stafford, & Hutchby, 2015).

Our chapter focuses on analysis of 28 mental health assessments, collected though a UK CAMH service. All families attending for initial assessments within the research time-frame of 6 months were approached, and consenting families were video-recorded for research purposes. Urgent referral and acute cases were excluded for clinical reasons. These assessments were multi-disciplinary in nature, and thus the format they took was not informed by a specific disciplinary framework. These practitioners included consultant, staff-grade and trainee child and adolescent psychiatrists, clinical psychologists, assistant psychologists, occupational therapists, community psychiatric nurses (CPNs) and psychotherapists. The children and young people were assessed by a minimum of two mental health practitioners (apart from in one case), and all 29 members of the clinical team participated.

The assessments generally lasted 90 minutes and the data corpus consisted of 2240 minutes in total. The demographics of the participants in the sample were 64% boys and 36% girls. The mean age was 11 years, ranging from 6 to 17 years. Usually children and young people attended with one or both of their parents (legal guardians), but in some cases also attended with siblings, members of the extended family and/or other professionals.

Analytic Approach

Understanding the nuances and subtleties of how children's competence is negotiated, navigated and treated, requires an analytic approach that explores how this is intersubjectively achieved through social interaction rather than objectively agreed. As noted earlier, for our interrogation of the data we utilised CA. This approach has been used extensively for analysing medical settings exploring interactions occurring between patients and their doctors in physical health settings (Robinson & Heritage, 2006; Stivers, 2002). Furthermore, CA has proven popular in mental health interactions because of its focus on the sequential order of talk and the social actions achieved by the range of parties (Heritage & Maynard, 2006; O'Reilly & Lester, 2017).

CA focuses on talk-in-interaction by examining the ways that talk is ordered and performs social actions (Hutchby & Wooffitt, 2008) and is an observational science in the sense that analysis is based on directly observable features in the data, showing that conversations are patterned, organised and stable (Drew, Chatwin, & Collins, 2001). This is particularly useful for the examination of mental health interactions because of its use of data that is yielded from real-world institutional interactions (Kiyimba, Lester, & O'Reilly, 2019). The use of naturally occurring data is favoured as it enables the analyst to capture what actually happens in real-world practice rather than retrospective reports, typically generated from interviews or focus groups (Kiyimba et al., 2019; Potter, 2002). This use of naturally occurring data is helpful for those practising CA, as analysts identify interactional practices in situ, so that recurrent and systematic patterns might be extracted (Drew et al., 2001). By focusing on these institutional interactions, a corpus of fragments can be generated to identify the recurrent sequential patterns within the talk and these are evidenced through the data and via co-analysis from multiple members which promotes rigour and objectivity (O'Reilly, Kiyimba, & Karim, 2016). Thus, our approach in this chapter is that of a collaborative partnership between academics and clinical-academics to promote translation of applied research into practice (O'Reilly & Kiyimba, 2015). The team-based approach to analysis, and input from the clinical author, ensures that the application of the CA to the clinical environment is meaningful and understandable to those practising in the field. In this way, a team-based approach to CA facilitates the translation of research to practise ensuring its impact.

For appropriate representation of the interactions within the initial mental health assessments, the Jefferson technique of transcription was utilised. This approach to transcription is a detailed technique that includes representing intonation, pauses and volume (Hepburn & Bolden, 2017; Jefferson, 2004).

Ethics

The sensitivity of the data, the nature of its collection and the potential vulnerability of the population meant that a stringent approach to ethics was utilised by the team. As the data were collected through the National Health Service (NHS), it was mandatory to undergo the standardised ethics process through the National Research Ethics Service and approval to undertake the project was provided. Mental health practitioners provided consent and facilitated approaching families. Families and children provided informed consent/assent together both before and after the assessment, and at both times were assured of their right to withdraw. Children and young people were provided with age-appropriate information sheets and had an opportunity to ask questions about the process. During the process of transcription pseudonyms were utilised to maintain anonymity and data were protected through encryption software.

An Analysis of Children and Young People's Social Competence

Children and young people's competence in mental health settings is a co-constructed endeavour, with each party having different degrees of access to specific epistemic domains. Broadly, these kinds of epistemic domains consist of adult–child, practitioner-lay and practitioner-personal expertise. In other words, the child and family are acknowledged to have access to an arena of knowledge situated within the personal domain of experiences, feelings, thoughts, behaviours and so on. However, practitioners are recognised as having a domain of knowledge situated within training, expertise, qualifications and clinical experience. Specifically, in the context of work with populations typically constructed by society as having less than full competence (e.g. children, the elderly, those with severe mental illness), the concept of 'half-membership' has been proposed as an explanatory framework for the differential rights to interactional involvement (Shakespeare, 1998).

The notion of half membership is a term that relates to the ways in which certain speakers are regarded as having full rights to speaking at any point in the interaction (full membership), whereas other speakers are restricted to having lesser rights to contribute (half membership). For example, children are frequently treated as having lesser rights to contribute to adult–child interactions than their adult counterparts (Hutchby & O'Reilly, 2010). It is acknowledged that there has been a conscious shift in policies and practices, with the advent of children's rights (UNCRC, 1989), and a drive for healthcare practices to be more child centred (Sőderback, Coyne, & Hardy, 2011). This reflects a new polemic of the sociology of children and childhood, constructing them as agents in their own lives (Corsaro, 2011). However, it is arguably still the case that in some healthcare interactions there have been cases whereby children in the conversation were treated by adults as having less competence to contribute than other adult speakers. The disparity between members' competences is additionally polarised in mental health adult and child interactions, whereby the adult has a specific domain of expertise and the child is more vulnerable by virtue of their potential mental health difficulty.

One arena of action where this additional polarisation of the disparity between members' competencies is identified, is within the mental health assessment. Compared to other arenas of actions where children and young people socially interact, such as in family groups or with peers, the institutional arena of action presents certain constraints on how their social competence is situated (Hutchby & Moran-Ellis, 1998). Within the institutional agenda of mental health assessments, competence is situated within a framework where interlocutors are provided with certain types of conversational opportunities or spaces, but not others. Often these opportunities to engage in the conversation for children and young people are restricted to answering specific questions by the mental health practitioner and only when addressed directly. Such interactional rights afforded to the child or young person are additionally imbued with institutional parameters of both the setting and the kinds of answers that are positioned as acceptable (Kiyimba, O'Reilly, & Lester, 2019). As such, the institutional space constrains the kinds of social competencies that can be displayed.

Previous research on problem presentation in mental health demonstrates that this phase of the appointment is a substantial part of the assessment process (O'Reilly et al., 2015). Understanding of the problem and history taking of family and developmental history are just some of the components that are fundamental to problem elicitation. Previous research has focused on children's understanding of their attendance at a mental health assessment, using this same data corpus, to specifically identify responses to a question asking, 'do you know why you are here?'. Notably, while some provided a possible mental health reason, most initially claimed insufficient knowledge with phrases such as 'I don't know'; although further analysis of the problem presentation phase indicated most children and young people were able to provide some account, whether pseudo-technical or lay, when the issue was further explored (Stafford, Hutchby, Karim, & O'Reilly, 2016).

The Core Sequence

The negotiation and testing of children and young people's social competence in the data analysed were constrained by the institutional setting and the assessment agenda. What was observed, however, were some regularities in the turn-taking structure of these sessions. Specifically, there was a recurring sequence of phases of interaction within the 'problem presentation' stage of the appointment:

- Phase one: Practitioner display of anticipated competence—typically the practitioner asked a question. The question focused on either the child/young person's understanding of why they were attending the assessment or their understanding of the reported problem.
- Phase two: The child or young person provided a candidate diagnosis in pseudo-technical language—often offering an immediate diagnostic label but in other cases, there was some hesitancy in explaining attendance at the assessment.
- Phase three: The practitioner 'tested' their competence in using the diagnostic label—this was done through a series of follow-up questions serving to elicit additional detail about behaviour and/or symptoms.
- Phase four: Demonstration by the practitioner of acceptance/rejection of the competence of the child/young person's response.

To illustrate the analytic focus, we present four detailed fragments of data. In the following first fragment, the young person was asked early in the session for a displayed understanding of his reasons for attending the assessment.

Fragment 1: Family 2

In this fragment, a 15-year-old male young person (YP) attended the assessment with his mother. Three clinical practitioners were present, although one was taking notes rather than participating. The outcome of the assessment was that the clinical team would seek out drug and alcohol services for the young person and some support work for the family if needed. We identify the phases of the sequence on the left side of the fragment with an arrow and corresponding phase number and embolden the text within the fragment to illuminate the key part of the turn.

Therapist	Um ↑do you ↑know (0.9) why you're here ↓tod↑ay?
	((looks at the YP))
	(0.8)
→1	**Can you tell me a bit ab↓out that?**
→2 YP	(Er) **it's ab↓out self-↓harmin'**.
Therapist	Ab↑out self-↓harm.
	(0.6)
	Ok↓a:y
	(1.8)
→3	i- and **what do you mean by ↓that Call↑um °in what**
	way°
YP	What (0.4) em: (0.4) it's (mainly) ↓I self-harm
Therapist	You self-↓harm
	(1.0)
	°okay° (.) c- can you say s↑omething about that ↓is
	it i- **↓do you cut yourself ↓or hurt yourself in a**
	↑different way?
YP	Cut
Therapist	↑You ↓cut yourself?
	(1.1)
	Is it on your ↑ar↓ms?
YP	((*YP nods*))
Therapist	°Okay,°
	(0.7)
	and **do you (0.3) need (0.6) stitches for that?**
YP	((*YP shakes head*))
→4 Therapist	°Okay°.
	(2.6)
	I'm gonna ↑ask you a bit about ↓that how ↑how long
	have you been doing ↓that ↑fo:r?
YP	About s↓even months.

This fragment is a straightforward example of how competence in using pseudo-technical language to describe the problem was, first, tested and then accepted by the mental health practitioner. The four phases of the sequence are evident here, as the social competence of the young person was negotiated. The practitioner opened the problem presentation part of the assessment with the commonly used question '↑*do you* ↑*know (0.88) why you're here* ↓*tod*↑ *ay?*', followed by '*Can you tell me a bit ab*↓ *out that*'. This demonstrated a display of anticipated competence (phase one of our sequence), first by presupposing that the young person may or may not know why they were there, but also by addressing him directly, rather than turning to the accompanying adult for information. By selecting the young person as the next speaker using 'you' and through eye gaze (Sacks, Schegloff, & Jefferson, 1974), the therapist treated him as potentially in possession of relevant knowledge to answer the question.

The young person's response '*it's ab*↓ *out self-*↓ *harming*' was presented in pseudo-technical language, thus forming the second phase of the sequence. He presented a candidate diagnosis in a factual way rather than a list of symptoms or characteristics consistent with the possible condition. In adult medical interactions, a more typical response to questions like 'why are you here?' is for the adult patient to describe several symptoms and provide space for the medical expert to develop a diagnosis (Ten Have, 1991). It may therefore be that the way in which young people present candidate diagnoses in factual ways, explains why practitioners test out the validity of this through a subsequent series of questions about symptoms and behaviours.

In presenting the candidate diagnosis the young person provided both a direct answer to the question, as well as recognising the institutional framework within which the question was asked, and also oriented to the kinds of language appropriate to that setting. In this way, the response indicates competence in several ways: first, that they can articulate the nature of the problem; second, they orient to the situated nature of the question, i.e. the person asking the question and the setting in which it was asked; third, that they can use the kind of institutional language relevant to the setting. The competence of the young person to attend to all of those facets of the interaction is quite a sophisticated communicative accomplishment.

The third phase of the sequence (the practitioner's displayed 'test' of competence) occurred over a series of turns:

what do you mean by ↓that Call↑ um °in what way° (line 10)
↓do you cut yourself ↓or hurt yourself in a ↑different way? (line 16/17)
Is it on your ↑ar↓ms (line 21)
do you (0.3) need (0.6) stitches for ↓that? (line 25)

Each of these incremental questions probed the young person's understanding of the meanings they ascribed to their initial response. This functioned to ascertain the behaviours the young person was engaged in that might fit with the clinical definition, in this case self-harming. The practitioner offered category-bound descriptors of behaviours (see Potter, 1996) that are congruent with the definition of self-harming. These questions worked as prompts regarding the types of answers being sought. The practitioner appears to be seeking confirmation or disconfirmation that the young person is competent to use the phrase self-harm in a clinically appropriate way. The minimal responses following each question are affirmative that their definition of the behaviours consistent with self-harm is the same as the practitioner's understanding.

The acknowledgement token '*okay.*' with a unit final intonation served as a transition point from the series of questions regarding the behaviours constituting self-harm, to signal a topic shift. Thus, the fourth phase of the sequence (demonstrated acceptance/rejection) in this instance is a degree of acceptance of the sufficiency of the young person's use of the phrase self-harm in what we are arguing to be a clinically sufficient way to indicate to the practitioner that the young person has competence to use the diagnostic category appropriately. Therefore, at this point there appears to be no requirement for the practitioner to pursue further information to clarify the young person's competent use of the diagnostic term. Additionally, there was a presupposition within the question '*↑how long have you been doing ↓that ↑fo:r?*' whereby the '*that*' indexically related back to the self-harming behaviour as having been interactionally agreed and provided a shared platform for further exploration.

Fragment 2: Family 12

In this fragment, the child is a 9-year-old female who attended the assessment with her mother. Three clinical practitioners were present during the assessment although again, one was only taking notes. The outcome of the assessment was that the child required treatment for anxiety and was referred for cognitive behaviour therapy.

Fragment 2

→1 Nurse	**I'd like it if you could tell me:(0.2) why you think**
	you've come here to↓day?
→2 Child	°Um: well **because I've got a phobia** but°
	((*child looks at mum*))
Mother	Just explain you you say K[ohm]
Child	° [what (d]o you me-) I
	don't know what she me:ans°
Nurse	You said you just said that you've come here because
	of your ↓phobia,
	(0.3)
→3	Okay **can you tell me a little bit more about**
	↑that?
Child	°Er:::°
	(2.0)
	°<We:ll I faint or I be sick when I see ↓needles
	or: blood or,>°
Nurse	Okay,
	(0.6)
	so (0.3) **you feel quite ↓faint (0.5) and sometimes**
	you're sick (0.3) if you see:(0.3) needles or blood
Mother	And she has actually ↓fainted
Nurse	**And you've actually ↓fainted**
Mother	Yeah
→4 Nurse	Okay.
	(1.4)
	↑how long's this been going on for?
Child	Er::m: since I's about (0.7) three.

This fragment consists of the same four phases of the identified sequence, in a way that demonstrates that the child's competence to adequately define the proposed problem was treated as sufficient. Here, the practitioner displayed an anticipation of competence from the child (phase one), by asking the question '*I'd like it if you could tell me: (0.2) why you think you've come here to↓day?*' This anticipated competence was displayed first, by directly addressing the child despite the mother's presence and the child's relatively young age. Second, by framing the question in terms of what 'you think', it projected the possibility of a range of potentially appropriate responses from the child's perspective. Subsequently, the child provided a pseudo-technical response '*because I've got a phobia*', which relates to phase two of the presented sequence. Like Fragment 1, this response was apparently then tested by the practitioner through a series of questions (phase three), such as '*can you tell me a little bit more about ↑that*' and reflections on the child's descriptions of phobia-congruent behaviour, '*so (0.3) you feel quite ↓faint*'. During these pursuit sequences in both fragments, the use of the token 'okay' (Fragment 1, line 23; Fragment 2, line

17), with continuing intonation and the short pause, signals that the pursuit is incomplete. In contrast, the sufficiency of the child's description (phase four) was signalled with the acknowledgement token '*okay.*' delivered with unit final intonation and a subsequent topic shift (Fragment 1, lines 27 and 29; Fragment 2, lines 25 and 27). The topic shift pursued detail, thus displaying a validation of the appropriateness of the child's answer.

Although the child in this fragment was considerably younger than the young person in the previous fragment, the practitioner directed their questions to the child, using speaker selection strategies to do so. This is especially notable, as the mother in this sequence was part of the conversation. There are two key points in the sequence where the mother jointly produced an explanation of the problem with the child. The first instance was a response to an invitation by the child, evidenced by the incomplete turn '*but...*' (line 3) and the child's eye gaze in the mother's direction, where the mother encouraged the child with a shortened version of her (pseudonym) name Kohemi (Kohm). The second instance was a self-initiated turn insertion by the mother '*she has actually ↓fainted*' (line 21) into a sequence between the practitioner and the child. Notably, despite interjection by the mother the practitioner still oriented their questions towards the child.

The social competence of the child in this sequence was oriented to by both the practitioner and the mother. The practitioner maintained her focus on the child using 'next-speaker selection' techniques, consequently treating the child as an agent competent to provide answers to specific questions. Furthermore, a degree of social competence was afforded to the child by the mother, as the mother actively agreed with the child's responses. She also gave space for the child to answer, even where there was a transition relevance place (Sacks et al., 1974) where she could speak, (i.e. the 2.0 pause). However, at the point where the practitioner downgraded the child's description of phobia-congruent behaviour from a clear action '*I faint or I be sick when I see ↓needles or: blood*', to a feeling state '*you feel quite ↓faint (0.5) and sometimes you're sick*', the mother interjected with a repair. In this case, she upgraded the practitioner's downgrade back to a behaviour rather than a feeling, using the discursive resource 'actually', '*she has actually ↓fainted*'. This may be indicative of the point at which the mother deemed the child's competence within the interaction not to be sufficiently developed to be able to challenge an adult who is in a position of authority. Thus, the mother did not allow enough floor space for the child to provide further detail. Compared to her previous demonstration of presumed competence of the child to answer questions about their own mental state directly, this interaction may be an assertion of her full membership as an adult in the interaction (Hutchby & O'Reilly, 2010).

Evidently therefore this fragment demonstrates a subtle difference from Fragment 1 in terms of membership status of the child. Here, the turns of the mother served an important role in the construction of the competence of the child. This was achieved by projecting anticipated competence for the child to answer the practitioner questions for herself at certain points and interjecting at other points where she treated the child as not competent to challenge the practitioner. This demonstrates that the notion of competence is not a binary construct but is something that is collaboratively, dynamically and situationally achieved.

Challenging and Testing Children's Competence

The fragments analysed thus far were straightforward examples of the ways in which competence was displayed with regard to why the child and the young person were attending the assessment appointment. In both cases, the practitioner displayed an anticipation of competence of the child/young person to answer questions about their mental health and a candidate diagnosis was provided. Although this understanding of the proposed diagnosis was apparently 'tested' and pursued by the practitioner, in both cases it was quite quickly confirmed and accepted. However, this is not always so straightforward, and we turn now to cases where the challenging and testing were more protracted and the confirmation not as readily forthcoming.

Fragment 3: Family 1

In this fragment, a 13-year-old female (YP) attended the assessment with her mother. Two clinical practitioners were present during the assessment. The outcome of the assessment was that further diagnostic work was required, to confirm a probable combination of anxiety disorder and Obsessive-Compulsive Disorder (OCD), and the team thus recommended a referral for diagnosis and treatment through CAMHS.

→1 Clin Psy	**↑Do you kno:w (0.3) why you've c↑ome here**
	toda↓y?
YP	Erm because (0.4) I- keep (0.9) doin' my-(0.4)
→2	**I thi↑nk it's ↓O- C- D-.**
Clin Psy	Ri:ght
	(0.8)
	↑Okay:
	(0.9)
	Um (0.5) °that is a (.) important word you use° (.)
	m↑eaning when you say O- C- D-,
YP	°Pard[on-]°
→3 Clin Psy	[ah] wh- **when you say o- c- d- what does**
	it me:an?
Mother	Wha' d'ya think it me:ans when you say o- c- d-?
YP	Um-
	(1.1)
	Ah: can't remember what the teacher to↑ld me=
Mother	=obsessive [compuls]ive disord[er
Clin Psy	[don't worry]
YP	[yeah that's it-
Clin Psy	er- right so you're ↑teacher told you that you
	may ↓ha:ve (.) obsessive c- compulsive disorder
Lines omitted	
Clin psy	**D↑o you mi↑nd just telling us a little mo:re** (0.5)
	er- w↑hat made the teacher sa:y that you ha↓ve (0.4)
	o- c- d?
YP	Because when I explained to her what I been doing
	she thought that that means li:ke (0.8) you get in
	like- a-(0.7) repe:ating the method and to keep
	do↑in' i↓t
Clin Psy	R:igh[t.
YP	[A::h
Mother	No but how did she notice that you got it?
	(0.5)
	coz you kept (0.4) cr[yin'
YP	[DOing it in no I's doin it in
	cla- when I's speaking to her I kept doing it (0.4)
	like (.) with the letters an' I'll do 'em.
Clin Psy	Ye:ah (0.5) °ehh° (0.6) **do you mind just telling**
	me what what do you [do you do
YP	[ah- every lette:r (.) thi:s is
	(.) going a bit now this one but- now [another
	on]e's coming
Clin Psy	[uh hum]
YP	↑This one (0.5) the ↑one befo:r↓e was l↑ike (0.81)
	>goin' on about< (0.7) letters that are for my
	fami>ly< (0.3) S for my mum L for my sister (0.5) K
	for my brother (0.4) D for my d↑ad
Clin Psy	Ri:ght,
YP	No M for my dad so[rry
Clin Psy	[Yea[h
YP	[then D for me (.) but I
	thought *((clears throat))* (0.8) now its c↓omin' I
	say ME at everythin'
Clin Psy	Ri::g[ht,
YP	[so if any I think things bad are g↓onna
	happen to my f↑amily so I'd r↓ather it happened to
	me-
→4 Clin Psy	**°Oka:y.°**
	(1.2)
	↑I'm so↓rry to h↑ear tha↓t

In this fragment, the young person offered up a candidate diagnosis of OCD (phase two of the proposed sequence) in response to the practitioner's display of anticipated competence (phase one of the proposed sequence). In the same way, as the previous two fragments, she offered a fairly direct response to the question, although this was hedged with '*I think*' which softened the projected factuality of the claim. The initial responses from the young person and mother to the practitioner's questioning about what OCD means, '*when you say o- c- d- what does it me:an?*' related to the specifics of the abbreviation, rather than the meaning of the condition itself.

14	Mother	Wha' d'ya think it me:ans when you say o- c- d-?
15	YP	um-
16		(1.1)
17		Ah: can't remember what the teacher to↑ld me=
18	Mother	=obsessiv[e compuls]ive disord[er
19	Clin Psy	[dont worry]

Here, the mother reframed the question from the practitioner in a way that allowed for a greater range of possible answers and positioned the knowledge in the domain of the young person, '*what d'ya think*'. In this way, the mother constructed the child as a 'competent conversational member', by providing conversational floor space, and presenting the question in a child-centred way, thus allowing for a forthcoming response (see Leiminer & Baker, 2000). When the young person was unable to recall the teacher's explanation of the abbreviation, the mother offered up the correct name of the condition. The '*don't worry*' response from the practitioner was indicative that central concern was not with the abbreviation, but the symptoms and behaviours associated with the condition.

What we see here is a range of potential competencies negotiated in the interaction; these are both projections from the practitioner and mother of anticipated competence in the young person, and displays of the young person's competence. As previously stated, competence is dynamically accomplished turn-by-turn throughout these data. In Fragment 3, there are several:

- Projected competence of the young person to comment appropriately on her reasons for attendance from the practitioner ↑*Do you kno:w (0.3) why you've c↑ome here toda↓y?* (lines 1–2).
- A display of competence from the young person to provide an institutionally appropriate response, in this case in the form of a pseudo-technical construct *I thi↑nk it's ↓O- C- D-* (line 4).
- A projected competence that the young person will be able to unpack the meaning of OCD from both the practitioner and the mother *Wha' d'ya think it me:ans when you say o- c- d-?* (line 14).
- A projected competence of the young person to articulate the reasons why the teacher attributed behaviours to OCD *w↑hat made the teacher sa:y that you ha↓ve (0.4) o- c- d-* (lines 24/25).
- A (partial) competence displayed by the young person in providing an explanation of this, though pursued by further questioning from the practitioner *Because when I explained to her what I been doing* (line 26).
- A (fuller) competence was displayed by the young person in the provision of descriptions of the behaviours and cognitions that are congruent with OCD *every lette:r .... S for my mum L for my sister* (lines 40–51).
- The practitioner treated the young person as having competently answered the question fully °*oka:y.*°*(1.2)*↑*I'm so↓rry to h↑ear tha↓t* (lines 58–60).

What is demonstrated here is that the acceptance of the young person's competence to express the behaviours and symptoms that map onto their initial candidate diagnosis was accomplished over a protracted series of turns. Thus, the young person was able to sustain a consistent narrative overextended turns of talk, which further evidences their competence in providing a more holistic overview of the issues, as well as attending to the practitioner's request for more information (*D↑o you mi↑nd just telling us a little mo:re;* and *do you mind just telling me what what do you do you do*). In institutional terms, the practitioner who is in an epistemic position to officially either accept or reject the candidate diagnosis requires a certain kind of information to inform that decision. The kinds of information required by the practitioner are: details about the type of problem, the recency and longevity of the symptoms and the seriousness of those symptoms and related behaviours. It appears that conversations about potentially problematic behaviours have already been engaged in prior to the assessment consultation between the young person, parents and third parties such as teachers. This fragment indicates that these conversations about behaviour have resulted in a lay-diagnosis of OCD being proposed prior to the assessment appointment. Therefore, when the young person presented a summation of these conversations at the outset of the assessment by stating a candidate diagnosis of OCD, the practitioner 'unpacked' the meaning of this label by questioning her further about her behaviour.

Fragment 4: Family 6

In this fragment, the child was a 9-year-old female who attended the assessment with her adoptive mother. Two clinical practitioners were present during the assessment. The outcome from this appointment was that the child did not have a mental health condition, and therefore, CAMHS was not the appropriate service. The team recommended parenting support for the mother.

Doctor	So when you ↓said that you were going to take a
	↓knife to yourself
	(1.0)
	Yeah
	(1.2)
→1	**What were you ↓hoping would happen?**
Child	Erm
	(2.5)
→2	**f::or me to ↓actually kill my↓self**
Doctor	Mummy w↑ould
Child	No me ↓to kill ↓myself
Doctor	Say that ↓again mummy would
Mum	↓No for her to kill her↓self
→3 Doctor	**Ri:ght you're ↑smiling as you ↓say that which makes**
	me ↓think that (.) was that really ↓some- ↓what you
	wanted to ↓do was kill yours↓elf?
Child	When I'm ang↓ry
	(1.7)
	I ↓do.
→4 Doctor	**And how long does that ↓last for ↓wanting to kill**
	yourself?
Child	Five m↓inutes.
Doctor	Umhm,
	(1.0)
	It's quite a g- good way of up↓setting ↑mum as ↑well
	isn't ↓it?
	(1.1)
Doctor	So if you're cross with ↓mum (.) and you say you're
	gonna kill your↓self (1.06) quite a way of ↓getting
	mum to kind of stop doing whatever she was doing
	that makes you ↑cross ↑isn't it?
	(1.6)
Child	((*nods head*))

Doctor	↑um (1.0) and then what ↓happens?
Child	°just g↓ive up°
Doctor	But I guess one of the ↓things it does ↓Carla is it
	kind of makes things ↑difficult for you and ↓mum
	because mum then ↓doesn't know what to ↑do with ↓you
	does ↓she?
	(0.9)
Doctor	Cuz you're not really what you're ↓saying to me is
	you're really kill ↓wanting to kill >your↓self<
	cause your cross
	(0.5)
	Yeah?
	(0.5)
Doctor	and you're cross with other people (0.5) but you're
	not really ↓wanting to di:e ↓if it only lasts five
	minutes ↑see what I'm getting ↓at
	(0.8)
	↑Okay
Child	((*nods head*))
	(1.0)
Doctor	**↑What do you ↑think might be a ↑different ↓way of**
	managing your feel↓ings cause (.) you're not it
	sounds to ↓me like you get ↓cross (0.5) yeah?
	(0.9)
	and you're not very ↓good at handling being
	↓cross

The four phases of the sequence are again clearly identified in this example. Of importance here, however, is that the fourth phase, namely accepting or rejecting the competence of the child, is more protracted and developed than in our previous fragments.

This fragment opens with the practitioner using the 'you said x' marker to introduce a prior topic using 'reflected speech' (see Kiyimba & O'Reilly, 2018). This device was shown to be effective in reintroducing sensitive topics with children (ibid.); in this case, the child's claim to '*take a ↓knife*' to herself. Significantly, however, it has also been shown to presage scepticism regarding the claims of an interlocutor (Hutchby, 1992). Once the receipt token 'yeah' had been received, the practitioner continued with the follow-up question, '*What were you ↓hoping would happen?*'. In this instance, the child's response was to emphatically assert that her hoped-for outcome would be '*f::or me to ↓actually kill my↓self*'. Interestingly, the child utilised the modal subjunctive 'actually' which has as one linguistic function, that of reinforcing the 'truth value' of the clause in which it appears (Clift, 2001; Quirk, Sidney, Leech, & Svartvik, 1985). It may be, therefore, that in projecting the need for such a definitive assertion about what she was *hoping* to happen, the child displayed interactional as well as linguistic competence in orienting to the potential scepticism in the practitioner's question.

The practitioner seemed to experience difficulty in hearing this assertion, despite its emphatic production; instead of attributing an outcome of the action with the knife upon the child herself, the turns '*Mummy w↑ould*' and '*Say that ↓again mummy would*' display an orientation to its intended effect upon the mother. Following repair of this mishearing, phase four of the sequence can be clearly seen, but in terms of both accepting and simultaneously rejecting aspects of the competence of the child, which was complex and subtly played out.

There is some evidence of partial acceptance through the practitioner's acknowledgement token, 'right'. There was a clear challenge from the practitioner questioning the validity of the child's answer in '*was that really ↓some- ↓what you wanted to ↓do*', which may also have been a challenge to the child's competence to 'correctly' identify their motivation. The addition of the word 'wanted' in the practitioner's challenge also reformulated the question from one focused on outcome to motivation. In terms of anticipated competence, several interrelated and nuanced aspects of the child's competence were presumed in this question:

1. Epistemically it was presumed that only the child herself could access her feelings and motivations.
2. To present this description of her feelings in response to a question, there was a competence required for the child to recognise her own internal state.
3. In recognising her internal state, a competence was needed to articulate and report on it to the practitioner.

The child's response was equally as emphatic in its assertion, '*I ↓do*' even though it was presented with the caveat, '*when I'm ang↓ry*'. In producing this account, what was demonstrated by the child was a competence regarding the recognition and reporting of her feelings and motivations for her actions. This competence was not challenged directly by the practitioner. Instead, and in line with the potential scepticism encoded in the earlier 'you said x' formulation, there was a suggestion that there may be additional functions to the described behaviour, such as '*up↓setting*

↑mum' and '*↓getting mum to kind of stop doing whatever she was doing that makes you ↑cross*'. Although the practitioner did not afford the child much opportunity to provide full or alternative responses, acknowledgement was indicated by the child with non-verbal agreement that provided the practitioner the opportunity to pursue this line of reasoning. In so doing, there was a scaffolding of the child's original claim against the practitioner's reconstruction of the motivation for it, which cumulated in '*you're not really ↓wanting to di:e*'. Once agreement from the child was acquired, the practitioner moved to propose an alternative solution to how the child manages her anger, suggesting the child had insufficient competence to do so currently: '*you're not very ↓good at handling being ↓cross*'.

Summary and Discussion

In this chapter, we explored the social interactions between children and young people and mental health practitioners, in the context of initial mental health assessments. Using naturally occurring data in the form of video-recordings, we focused on the social competencies of the children and young people in these assessments. In response to a presupposition of competence to communicate issues and experiences of mental health, children and young people (in these examples) offered a candidate diagnosis. The focus of this chapter was to gauge the ways in which children and young people display and were treated as needing to display, competence in using institutionally relevant mental health discourses in problem presentation sequences.

Following the principles of unmotivated looking in CA (Sacks, 1984), the use of medicalised terminology and use of candidate diagnosis stood out as unusual. With closer attention paid to the broader literature and the fragments of data, it was observed that the adult interlocutors in these assessment interactions treated these responses as insufficient in their own right and as requiring further exploration. These pursuits typically took the form of seeking information about symptom and behaviour frequency and severity. Previous research examining paediatric clinics involving parents and children has shown that when parents offer a candidate diagnosis, they are treated by the doctor as taking a stance that seeks confirmation as the preferred response (Stivers, 2002: 308).

```
Doc:  Al:ri:ght, well what can I do [for you today.
Mom:                                [(°hm=hm=hm=hm.°)
Mom         .hhh Uhm (.) Uh- We're- thinking she might have an ear
            infection? [in thuh left ear?
Doc:                   [Okay,
```

Stivers reported that the offering of candidate diagnoses in these paediatric clinics tended to be tentative and heavily mitigated. In the fragment above, the use of words '*thinking*' and '*might*' from the mom, together with strong questioning intonation, served to highlight that the diagnosis was offered up for confirmation or disconfirmation. In our data, in contrast, when offering a candidate diagnosis, the children/young people did not engage in the same hedging or tentative proposals. Instead, they tended simply to present the candidate diagnosis with minimal or no mitigation.

We noted that the negotiation of competence was sequentially accomplished through a typical four-phase configuration. To summarise, this was, first a practitioner display of anticipated competence of the child or young person to respond to the question; second, the provision of a candidate diagnosis in pseudo-technical language by the child or young person; third, the testing of competence in terms of the congruence between the proposed label and the symptoms and behaviour reported; and fourth, an eventual display of accepting or rejecting the competence of that proposal. The ways in which this linguistic trajectory was built incrementally over a series of turns are important because the institutional task of these initial mental health assessments is primarily to determine whether the child or young person has an identifiable mental health problem that warrants an intervention from specialist CAMH services. Part of this determination involves an evaluation of the longevity and extremity of the symptoms and/or behaviours.

Rather than taking the child or young person's assertion of a diagnosis at face value during the problem presentation phase of the appointment, practitioners displayed further questioning sequences to establish what behaviours and symptoms had precipitated the asserted diagnosis.

This implies that the practitioner required more information to accept their competence to appropriately label the condition. Although this may project a rather binary conceptualisation of the notion of competence, our investigation of the data highlighted the more subtle and nuanced aspects of anticipated and displayed competence. Specifically, for an utterance to be treated as sufficiently competent, the preceding question had to be positioned as seeking an answer which would be within the child or young person's epistemic domain. In these cases, questions about the nature of the problem or reasons for attendance were treated as within their domain to answer. The answers provided were treated as displaying competence with regard to using appropriate language for the institutional setting, but not necessarily in the format that adults would typically present their responses in this context.

The child or young person's epistemic domain was treated as one of intrapersonal thoughts, feelings and motivation, while the practitioner's epistemic domain was in clinical knowledge, expertise and understanding of how behaviours and symptoms relate to diagnostic labels or mental ill health symptom clusters. Predominantly, the data indicate that the practitioners were not challenging the epistemics of the child/young person in terms of their feelings, thoughts and behaviours, but instead were testing the boundaries of that domain at the place where it intersected with the practitioner's epistemic domain of knowledge about mental health.

The practitioner cannot be expected to know about the child/young person's feelings or thoughts, and neither can they be expected to know about their life at home; however, the practitioner is an expert in a different area, that is, the clinical one. While the child/young person's thoughts and feelings may be treated by practitioners as personal knowledge, where there is an overlap between the child's and practitioner's epistemic domain (i.e. to determine 'correct labelling' of problematic behaviours, thoughts and feelings within a medicalised language), it is this area that is more likely to be treated as needing to be negotiated.

Conclusions

Evident from the analysis is the sophisticated and competent ways in which the children and young people attended to the institutional environment and the clinical encounter. Our analysis demonstrated that the practitioners oriented to the anticipated competence of the child or young person to provide satisfactory answers to questions about their attendance and the nature of the problem. These children and young people subsequently demonstrated interactional competence in many ways, such as answering questions in an appropriate and accepted manner, being able to articulate their thoughts, feelings and behaviours, and orienting to the institutional boundaries of the assessment interaction. As we have acknowledged, competence is not binary, and they were treated as having unquestioned competence in articulating certain aspects of knowledge, whereas more subtle competencies, such as their ability to use medical terminology 'correctly' were tested and explored. In effect, social competence can only be understood as something that is situated, contextualised and collaboratively achieved.

Professional Reflection

Nikki Kiyimba

Abstract

Nikki Kiyimba is a contributing author to the chapter and a Chartered Clinical Psychologist. She offers a clinical reflection on the value of using conversation analysis to inform practice and the core messages learned for child mental health practitioners from this chapter. In her reflection, she addresses the bidirectional influence of coming to a set of data as both a researcher and clinical practitioner. Trained as a conversational analyst, she is able to separate what the interactants might be 'intending' in a cognitive reductionist way and focus on the social actions in the data. As a practitioner, she is also able to step away from the transcripts and the analysis to see what the interactants are accomplishing in their talk and how they achieve it, and to think about what the implications might be to feed back into clinical work.

As a co-author on this project, it has been a really interesting experience to consider the bidirectional influence of coming to a set of data as both a researcher and clinical practitioner. When analysing the data, I still hold onto my roots as a discursive psychologist and my conversational analytic training that separates me from imagining what the interactants might be 'intending' or 'trying to do' in some kind of cognitive reductionist way. This allows me, along with my co-authors, to really see what the social actions are in the interaction and how they are developed turn-by-turn in a sequential order. Then as a practitioner, I can also step back from what the text shows that the interactants are accomplishing in their talk and how they achieve it, and to think about what the implications might be to feed back into clinical work. When I think particularly about children and young people's competence, the development of this chapter has been a real journey from a rather clunky binary perception of 'competent versus non-competent', when we first approached the data. It has developed into a far more meaningful appreciation for the sophisticated and nuanced nature of children's social competence, and a realisation that competence is displayed and co-constructed in a multitude of layers and subtle inflections.

What has been most inspiring, is to see in detail how a single turn of talk from a practitioner can contain within it several presuppositions about the different kinds of competencies that a child or young person would need to have in order to respond appropriately or adequately. Digging into the detail of the data and discussing it with my co-authors have unearthed interesting aspects that otherwise may not have been discovered. This is one of the great joys of academic collaboration, as new insights are borne through collaborative inquiry. The idea that there are actually a range of potential competencies that are negotiated within the interaction is one such enlightenment that emerged from these discussions. When working with children, as with adults, we all have degrees of competence in different areas and may be competent in one thing but totally incompetent in another. The exciting thing about conversation analysis is that we can see the moments in a dynamic, in-action conversation where particular kinds of competencies are projected and displayed. Not only are these dynamic, situated accomplishments, they are also fascinatingly co-constructed.

One example of this co-construction of competence was in Fragment 2 where the mother stepped in after having been taking a rather 'back stage' position in the exchange between the practitioner and the child. She quite assertively intervened with an interjection to upgrade the practitioner's comment, and in so doing backed up what the child had said, protecting the child's statement from being minimised by the practitioner. Where competence is assumed, unquestioned and is displayed fairly unproblematically, it can sometimes be more difficult to see than in those moments where something happens to disrupt the flow. This was one of those moments, where the mother displayed a moment of treating the child as having insufficient competence *in that moment, with that practitioner, in that setting*, to engage in a *particular kind* of competence. In this instance, the particular kind and degree of competence inferred as not yet developed might be something like the competence to assert herself in challenging the downgrade of the adult authority figure of the practitioner.

As with all research, I find that one of the outcomes of this kind of detailed inquiry is that it raises even more questions and other avenues for potential research. Another area that came to light was that the children in these data usually presented their candidate diagnosis quite directly and plainly stated. In our discussions as co-authors, we pondered on why this seemed different from our anecdotal experiences and understandings of adult interactions in similar kinds of medical situations. We started to muse on the fact that as adults, our experience tells us that when presented with a medical expert, we are more likely to present a series of symptoms and generally allow the 'expert' to come to a conclusion about what the sum of these parts might indicate. In effect, we as adults are more likely to offer the pieces of the jigsaw, but then (even if we have an idea of what we think the answer might be) defer to the medical practitioner to provide a definitive answer or 'diagnosis'. Might it be that the children and young people in these data just hadn't developed that level of social competence or familiarity with the script or schema for attending a medical appointment? Or might something else be at play? Conversation analysis has its roots in sociological enquiry and the work of Harvey Sacks, an academic interested in how people create their social world through words and interactions with others. These are just the kinds of questions that CA asks about how people talk to one another and accomplish social actions through their words.

As a practitioner, what I take away from this particular foray into the world of mental health assessments is a far greater appreciation and insight into the kinds of presuppositions embedded in any question that I may be asking a client. By asking any question of a client, I am on some level assuming various degrees and arenas of competence; be that the ability to think, to remember what I have said long enough to answer, to hear what I have said, to be able to understand the words I am speaking, to access their own thoughts or feelings, to be able to put some kind of linguistic label on those inner experiences and to have the confidence and will to speak to me and to articulate those experiences in a way that I can understand. Perhaps it does us all good from time to time to examine our own presuppositions about others' competencies and not assume too much … or too little.

References

Clift, R. (2001). Meaning in interaction: The case of actually. *Language, 77*(2), 245–291.

Corsaro, W. (2011). *The sociology of childhood* (3rd ed.). Thousand Oaks, CA: Pine Forge Press.

Danby, S. (2002). The communicative competence of young children. *Australian Journal of Early Childhood, 27*(3), 25–30.

Danby, S., & Baker, C. (1998). 'What's the problem?' Restoring social order in the preschool classroom. In I. Hutchby & J. Moran-Ellis (Eds.), *Children and social competence: Arenas of action* (pp. 157–186). London: Falmer Press.

Drew, P., Chatwin, J., & Collins, S. (2001). Conversation analysis: A method for research into interactions between patients and health-care practitioners. *Health Expectations, 4*(1), 58–70.

Hepburn, A., & Bolden, G. (2017). *Transcribing for social research.* London: Sage.

Heritage, J., & Maynard, D. W. (2006). Problems and prospects in the study of physician-patient interaction: 30 years of research. *Annual Review of Sociology, 32*(1), 351–374.

Hutchby, I. (1992). The pursuit of controversy: Routine scepticism in talk on "talk radio". *Sociology, 26*(4), 673–694.

Hutchby, I. (2007). *The discourse of child counselling.* Amsterdam: John Benjamins.

Hutchby, I., & Moran-Ellis, J. (1998). Situating children's competence. In I. Hutchby & J. Moran-Ellis (Eds.), *Children and social competence: Arenas of social action* (pp. 7–26). London: Falmer Press.

Hutchby, I., & O'Reilly, M. (2010). Children's participation and the familial moral order in family therapy. *Discourse Studies, 12*(1), 49–64.

Hutchby, I., & Wooffitt, R. (2008). *Conversation analysis* (2nd ed.). Oxford: Blackwell.

James, A., & Prout, A. (Eds.). (1990). *Constructing and reconstructing childhood: Contemporary issues in the sociological study of childhood.* London: Falmer Press.

James, A., & Prout, A. (1997). Re-presenting childhood: Time and transition in the study of childhood. In A. James & A. Prout (Eds.), *Constructing and reconstructing childhood: Contemporary issues in the sociological study of childhood* (2nd ed., pp. 230–250). Oxon: Routledge.

Jefferson, G. (2004). Glossary of transcript symbols with an introduction. In G. Lerner (Ed.), *Conversation analysis: Studies from the first generation.* Amsterdam: John Benjamins Publishing Company.

Karim, K. (2015). The value of conversation analysis: A child psychiatrist's perspective. In M. O'Reilly & J. N. Lester (Eds.), *The Palgrave handbook of child mental health: Discourse and conversation studies* (pp. 25–41). Basingstoke: Palgrave Macmillan.

Kiyimba, N., Lester, J., & O'Reilly, M. (2019). *Using naturally occurring data in qualitative health research: A practical guide.* Cham: Springer.

Kiyimba, N., & O'Reilly, M. (2018). Reflecting on what 'you said' as a way of reintroducing difficult topics in child mental health assessments. *Child and Adolescent Mental Health, 23*(3), 148–154.

Kiyimba, N., O'Reilly, M., & Lester, J. (2019b). Agenda setting with children using the three wishes technique. *Journal of Child Health Care, 22*(3), 419–432.

Leiminer, M. J., & Baker, C. D. (2000). A child's say in parent—Teacher talk at the pre-school: Doing conversation analytic research in early childhood settings. *Contemporary Issues in Early Childhood, 1*(2), 135–152.

Mackay, R. W. (1991). Conceptions of children and models of socialization. In F. C. Waksler (Ed.), *Studying the social worlds of children: Sociological readings* (pp. 23–37). London: Falmer Press.

Mash, E., & Hunsley, J. (2005). Special section: Developing guidelines for the evidence-based assessment of child and adolescent disorders. *Journal of Child and Adolescent Psychology, 34*(3), 362–379.
Mayall, B. (1994). Children in action at home and in school. In B. Mayall (Ed.), *Children's childhoods observed and experienced* (pp. 114–127). London: Falmer Press.
O'Reilly, M., Karim, K., & Kiyimba, N. (2015a). Question use in child mental health assessments and the challenges of listening to families. *British Journal of Psychiatry Open, 1*(2), 116–120.
O'Reilly, M., Karim, K., Stafford, V., & Hutchby, I. (2015b). Identifying the interactional processes in the first assessments in child mental health. *Child and Adolescent Mental Health, 20*(4), 195–201.
O'Reilly, M., & Kiyimba, N. (2015). *Advanced qualitative research: A guide to contemporary theoretical debates.* London: Sage.
O'Reilly, M., Kiyimba, N., & Karim, K. (2016). "This is a question we have to ask everyone": Asking young people about self-harm and suicide. *Journal of Psychiatric and Mental Health Nursing, 23,* 479–488.
O'Reilly, M., & Lester, J. (2017). *Examining mental health through social constructionism: The language of mental health.* Basingstoke: Palgrave.
Potter, J. (1996). *Representing reality: Discourse, rhetoric and social construction.* London: Sage.
Potter, J. (2002). Two kinds of natural. *Discourse Studies, 4*(4), 539–542.
Quirk, R., Sidney, G., Leech, G., & Svartvik, J. (1985). *A comprehensive grammar of English language.* London: Longman.
Robinson, J., & Heritage, J. (2006). Physicians' opening questions and patients' satisfaction. *Patient Education and Counselling, 60,* 279–285.
Sacks, H. (1984). Notes on methodology. In J. M. Atkinson & J. Heritage (Eds.), *Structures of social action: Studies in conversation analysis* (pp. 21–27). Cambridge: Cambridge University Press.
Sacks, H. (1995). *Lectures on Conversation* (2 Vols.). Oxford: Blackwell.
Sacks, H., Schegloff, E., & Jefferson, G. (1974). A simplest systematic for the organization of turn-taking for conversation. *Language, 50,* 696–735.
Sands, N. (2004). Mental health triage nursing: An Australian perspective. *Journal of Psychiatric Mental Health Nursing, 11,* 150–155.
Shakespeare, P. (1998). *Aspects of confused speech: A study of verbal interaction between confused and normal speakers.* Mahwah, NJ: Lawrence Erlbaum Associates.
Silverman, D. (1987). *Communication and medical practice.* London: Sage.

Sőderback, M., Coyne, I., & Harder, M. (2011). The importance of including both a child perspective and the child's perspective within health care settings to provide truly child-centred care. *Journal of Child Health Care, 15*(2), 99–106.

Stafford, V., Hutchby, I., Karim, K., & O'Reilly, M. (2016). 'Why are you here?' Seeking children's accounts of their presentation to CAMHS. *Clinical Child Psychology and Psychiatry, 21*(1), 3–18.

Stivers, T. (2002). Presenting the problem in pediatric encounters: "Symptoms only" versus "candidate diagnosis" presentations. *Health Communication, 14*(3), 299–338.

Ten Have, P. (1991). Talk and institution: A reconsideration of the 'asymmetry' of doctor–patient interaction. In D. Boden & D. Zimmerman (Eds.), *Talk and social structure*. Cambridge: Polity Press.

Theobald, M. (2016). Achieving competence: The interactional features of children's storytelling. *Childhood, 23*(1), 87–104.

United Nations. (1989). *Conventions on the rights of the child.* New York: UN.

3

The Social Organization of Echolalia in Clinical Encounters Involving a Child Diagnosed with Autism Spectrum Disorder

Michie Kawashima and Douglas W. Maynard

Professional Reflection by Tetsuya Abe

Introduction

Children with developmental disabilities face stigma and stereotyping from others in their lives, associated with their perceived incompetence in or inability to interact with others (Gray, 2002). *Echolalia*, which refers to the automatic repetition of words or phrases, is a characteristic speech

M. Kawashima (✉)
Department of International Studies, Kyoto Sangyo University, Kyoto, Japan
e-mail: a006374@cc.kyoto-su.ac.jp

D. W. Maynard
Department of Sociology, University of Wisconsin-Madison, Madison, WI, USA
e-mail: maynard@ssc.wisc.edu

J. Lamerichs et al. (eds.), *Children and Mental Health Talk*,
The Language of Mental Health,
https://doi.org/10.1007/978-3-030-28426-8_3

pattern of individuals who meet the diagnostic criteria of what is currently known as Autism Spectrum Disorder and are at risk for stigmatization and stereotyping (DSM 5th, 2013). Echolalia often presents in early childhood and is generally viewed as an indication of Autism Spectrum Disorder—particularly, as a symptom of the communication deficit—in clinical settings.

In this chapter, we examine whether echolalia as a speech pattern has different interactional functions depending on its sequential location in clinical conversations. We analyzed two videotaped clinical sessions between a child with Autism Spectrum Disorder and clinicians, which included several test batteries. We focused on how echolalia in the interaction between the child and professionals emerges within the standardized tasks that the child with Autism Spectrum Disorder had to perform.

The study concerns *immediate echolalia*, which refers to the child's repetition of a single phrase or sentence heard at that moment. This differs from *delayed echolalia*, or the repetition of past utterances, including those emitted in other settings than the current one. The analysis first examines how echolalia works conversationally within a turn-taking system. More specifically, it analyzes how echolalia operates within the instruction and testing sequences described by Marlaire and Maynard (1990) and Maynard and Marlaire (1992), which consist of three turns, as follows:

Teacher: What is this? Question (initiation)
Child: Apple. Answer (reaction)
Teacher: Good! Evaluation

The analysis is based on the perspective that echolalia relates to the completion of tasks in test batteries, in and through the "interactional substrate" (Marlaire & Maynard, 1990) of psychological testing, which is discussed later in this paper.

The second part of the analysis focuses on how echolalia contributes to a bodily action such as moving a piece in a puzzle, in that nonvocal activities are also considered to be an important aspect of the interactional substrate (Maynard & Marlaire, 1992), which functions as an essential basis for the possibility of testing. In order to analyze whether or how a child performs tasks in a testing sequence in which the child needs to comply with instructions requiring bodily actions, we examine how a clinician's utterances are intended to invite bodily action and how the child handles such invitations. Finally, we discuss how the analysis of echolalia can contribute to or aid the completion of tasks in a testing situation by a child with Autism Spectrum Disorder. That manifestation of echolalia fits with what Maynard and Turowetz (2017: 472) define as the realm of "concrete competence"—"the basic know-how or set of skills and practices required to participate in social activities," including formal ones, such as test-taking.

Previous Research

Fay (1969) defined immediate echolalia as the meaningless repetition of a word just spoken by another speaker. Delayed echolalia, on the other hand, involves repeating a phrase or sentence heard in a conversation at some earlier point in time. This latter type has been drawing the attention of researchers because it can be seen as one of the ways by which researchers can understand how individuals with Autism Spectrum Disorder "process information, organize their experiences, conceive of language and in some cases, attempt to participate in social exchange" (Schuler & Prizant, 1985: 164). As well, delayed echolalia is considered to be related to cognitive, memory, and other neuropsychological deficits. Immediate echolalia is often treated as an indication of language incomprehension (Fay, 1969; Shapiro, 1977). However, since immediate echolalia involves the repetition of utterances heard at that moment, it can indicate that the child is engaged with the current social exchange and is oriented toward the interaction. This behavior suggests that the child is exhibiting concrete competence. Our question is how immediate echolalia as interactional resources contributes to diagnostic testing circumstances.

The literature on Autism Spectrum Disorder has shown that echolalia generally serves positive functions in communication, especially when a recipient shows that they have "interpreted" the echolalic utterance (Prizant, 1978; Prizant & Duchan, 1981; Sterponi & Shankey, 2014; Tarplee & Barrow, 2009). Some studies have explored evidence of the interactional function and comprehension within immediate echolalic behavior (Prizant, 1978; Prizant & Duchan, 1981) and were able to identify several types of immediate echolalia based on its use: non-focused, turn-taking, declarative, rehearsal, self-regulatory, yes-answer, and request. This research indicates that echolalia can provide hints as to the competence of the child with Autism Spectrum Disorder, depending on the features of the echolalia.

Tarplee and Barrow (2009) conducted a case study on delayed echolalia using conversation analysis, seeking to identify how echolalia serves as an interactional resource. Their findings indicate that delayed echolalia helps establish intersubjectivity between a child with Autism Spectrum Disorder and mother. During interactions, delayed echolalia can solicit particular responses that carry routine and specific meanings for the participants.

However, Wootton (1999) has pointed out that, when engaged in delayed echoing, a child with Autism Spectrum Disorder may be disengaged communicatively from other people, even though the child is exhibiting an orientation to their interactional presence. That is, the child may position his echoes relative to segments such as turn boundaries in talk, suggesting a kind of monitoring of another's speech, but his echoes are otherwise non-interactional.

Using a detailed conversational and prosodic analytical approach, Sterponi and Shankey (2014) analyzed video recordings of a 5-year-old child with delayed and immediate echolalia in the home. They found that the child used both immediate and delayed echolalia with various modifications to the prosody as well as reformulations in order to steer interactions in a desired direction. For example, in response to directives, the child utilized immediate echolalia with marked modification to the prosodic contour to show his resistance. Sterponi and Shankey (2014) concluded that the echolalia enabled the child to express more nuance in his stance in an ongoing interaction.

Our study shares the view that echolalia serves as an interactional resource; also in fulfilling/completing certain institutional testing tasks. However, examination of immediate echolalia in an institutional setting (e.g., diagnostic testing) has not been fully studied in previous research. Therefore, it is relevant to determine where in conversation immediate echolalia occurs and the specific function of its placement in the context of the systematic evaluation of a child's ability.

Marlaire and Maynard (1990) noted that the testing sequence of an educational exam depends upon an "interactional substrate," which is established through collaborative work among participants. "The substrate consists of such practical activities as prompting with test items, answering, initiating repair and correction of prompts and answers, doing the repair and correction, acknowledging, evaluating, and engaging in other vocal and nonvocal embodied practices so as to effect the test as an official and valid enterprise" (Maynard & Marlaire, 1992: 193). This interactional substrate is therefore constructed through subtle cues from each participant—e.g., smiling, tone of voice, the form of third-turn responses—and acknowledgments from the clinician (Maynard & Marlaire, 1992). Echolalia may be one such subtle cue by the child and constitute one of the practical activities or forms of "concrete competence" (Maynard & Turowetz, 2017)—that sustain the interactional basis of the testing environment for the clinician and child.

Data and Methods

The data comprise two clinical sessions between a 5-year-old child with Autism Spectrum Disorder and clinicians videotaped in the mid-1980s. It comes from a larger data set involving 13 cases of children being evaluated in a US clinic for developmental disabilities. As Maynard and Turowetz (2017: 471) note, diagnostic tests, standards, and criteria have changed over time, but there has been an interactional organization that has remained stable over time; see also Maynard and Turowetz (2019). Hence, the data are part of a larger data set, and our selections were made because of the phenomena of echolalia they contain. Our analysis is something like the single episode analytic strategy that Schegloff (1987) espouses and illustrates, where past work in CA is utilized in the analytic explication of a singular fragment or singular aspects in a small fragment of talk. Each of our two sessions was approximately one hour in length. The first session was conducted by a special education clinician and comprised several test batteries employed to identify problems in the child's ability to learn. Each test battery included a series of sub-tests. For example, there was a puzzle completion task, which consisted of different kinds of puzzle with animals and people. The second session was a pediatrician's meeting with the same child and his parents and included physical exams and sensory tests.

We analyzed the data primarily using conversation analysis, as this allows for a detailed and precise description of the interactions among participants (Clayman & Gill, 2012; Heritage, 2005; Sidnell & Stivers, 2013). Conversation analysis ensures a rich description of the ongoing sequential organization manifested in social interaction. Using this methodology, we could focus precisely on which parts of the conversation are repeated by the child and how this repetition is handled by both parties during the testing situation. As such, a sequential examination of echolalia may help in characterizing how echolalia contributes to the testing setting.

Analysis

Within the data set, most of the conversation, as explained in Marlaire and Maynard (1990), takes the form of a testing sequence [initiating (question)—reply (answer)—evaluation], which is similar to the IRE sequence in educational settings (Mehan, 1985). The test results are determined by evaluating whether the child's reaction is what is expected in that particular sequence—a display of "abstract competence" or the ability to produce general answers to theoretical or empirical questions. Accordingly, when the child repeats the first turn of the testing sequence—that is, the question—it may be considered inappropriate or wrong as an answer, although it may incorporate other skills.

This study finds four main patterns of echolalia within the testing sequence. The first pattern of immediate echolalia involved the repetition of a prior question addressed to the person with echolalia. The second pattern involved the repetition of a question followed by the production of an answer to that question. The third pattern involved repeating questions a number of times. The last and fourth pattern has a similar structure to the third and involved repeating the assessment within assessment-agreement sequences. Across these patterns, there are a number of consistent features related to the turn-exchange system and embodied interaction.

Echolalia in Question–Answer Sequences

Below is an fragment from a conversation between the clinician and the child with Autism Spectrum Disorder. The child, whose pseudonym is Tony Smith, was 7 years and 9 months old when school personnel referred him to a diagnostic clinic in 1985—see Turowetz and Maynard (2017) for an investigation of the diagnostic proceedings for Tony. During one portion of the examination, the clinician ("C") and Tony ("T") sat obliquely at the same table. Each had a number of pieces of paper used to complete the "little boy puzzle." In the prior conversation, the clinician had suggested that the child put the pieces of paper together in the shape of a boy, as she proceeded to complete the puzzle on her own. Having finished putting these pieces into the shape of a boy, they began gluing them together on a base mat. In this fragment, Tony is trying to glue the boy's pants onto the mat.

Transcript Instruction

[()] = Bodily movement overlapping with utterance

(()) = Bodily movement without overlapping utterance

Fragment 1

```
    T: ((putting glue on the pants and giving the glue back to
       clinician))
    C: Thank you. Good for you.
    T: ((bringing the pants upside down on the paper and turning
       the pants around))
    C: Is that the way the pants go_
    T: (2.5)((putting the pants upside down on the paper))
 →  T: [Is sat the way pants go_ Ss. (0.8)
    T: [(Stopping the hand movement)]
    C: N::o, You put it in the way they go.
    T: (0.5)((starting to turn the pants around))
    C: Yeah. I know you know that's good.
    T: (1.5)((stops at the almost correct position, with slight smile))
    C: That's good.
    T: (2.0)((starts torqueing his body to look at clinician and smiles))
    C: All ri[ght.  Just okay o:::h.]
    C:       [(putting the hand around the pants piece)]
    T: ((tracking the clinician's hand movement, still with slight smile))
    C: Let's put him up here.
    T: ((placing the pants))
    C: ((pushing the pants piece on the paper with the child's hand))
```

In this interaction, the clinician formulated a question about how the pants should be oriented on the paper (line 6), when the child began to put the pants upside down (line 7). After turning the piece around again, in an echolalic way, the child repeated the clinician's question (line 8). Subsequently, on line 10, the clinician herself produced the answer to the question.

In this instance, the child repeated the clinician's initial question. Sacks, Schegloff, and Jefferson (1974) noted that questions, when positioned as the first part of an adjacency pair, set "a constraints on what should be done in the next turn" (i.e., answering; p. 719). That is, Tony is in the "second position" relative to the question as a "first position" utterance (Schegloff, 2007). He avoids the constraint to provide an answer by repeating the question, which in effect is a "counter" that changes the direction of the sequence.

Notice how, after answering the child with "no" (line 10), the clinician answered the question herself, which, in effect, encouraged Tony to produce the correct answer or move. When the question was initiated by the clinician (line 6), the child was holding the pants piece upside down (line 7). While repeating the question (line 8), the child stopped moving the piece (line 9). As the clinician answered her own question and directed Tony to "put it in the way they go" (line 10), the child began to relocate the piece (line 11). With the elicited encouragement from the clinician (line 12), and the child eventually reached a nearly correct position (line 13). Subsequently, the clinician gave the child a positive assessment (line 14). At this point, the child looks at the clinician with a slight smile (line 15).

Three points are of note here. First, the echolalia enabled a path for the child to avoid the social force of the question within the testing sequence, but without being heard as evasive or (more extremely) as leaving the interaction field (cf. Sacks 1989). That is, independently of producing an answer that could be coded as either correct or incorrect, Tony shows concrete competence (Maynard & Turowetz, 2017) in the sheer ability to produce an utterance in the answer "slot" of a testing sequence. Second, the echolalia elicited an instructional sequence of interaction within the testing sequence. Maynard and Marlaire (1992) noted that the instructional sequence is a preparatory phase of the interactional substrate that interactants often produce before entering the actual testing sequence. However, the authors do note that instruction can occur in the middle of the testing, and this is clearly evident in this case—the child received instruction on how to carry out the required task.

Third, with regard to bodily movement, the fragment shows the multimodal way in which the clinician directed the child, both haptically (via touch, line 9) and gesturally by handling the pants. This directive movement was received by the child positively, as evidenced by his smiling facial expression and compliance with the directive action. The clinician's instructional utterances further encouraged the child's completion of the task, which was needed for the appropriate evaluation. Completion of the task was therefore clearly marked by the collaborative action between both parties.

Echolalia with the Production of an Answer

Verbal alignment: When echolalia is located within a testing question-answer-evaluation sequence, it can be accompanied by an answering utterance that fulfilled the original sequential constraint of a testing question. This was evidenced in Fragment 2, which occurred just after Tony assumed that he had finished gluing of pieces onto the base of the "little boy" puzzle task.

Fragment 2

```
    C: You finish al:l by yourself.  That's a nice job.
    T: (8.0)((gluing & putting the piece on the paper))
    C: Okay.
    T: (4.0)((gluing & putting the piece on the paper))
    C: Ni::ce job.
    C: (1.5) Okay. An- (3.5)
    T: shu:
    T: (20.0)((putting other pieces on the paper))
    T: ((putting his hands off the paper and to the side)
       ((looking torward the camera with slight smile))
    C: Are you all do::ne? (1.2) We for[got one thing.]=
    T:                                 [(facing to the clinician)]
    C: =Can you find what we forget?
       (1.5)
    C: Ton[y, you forgot the one thing. ]
    T:    [(facing to the clinician and looking down at the paper)]
    C: What did we fo[rget? (0.8)]
    T:               [(start rocking and looking at the paper)]
    C: Look. [what did we forget? (4.0)]
             [(pushes the base paper close to Tony, picking
               up ear piece and putting it on the paper.)]
    T: ((rocking & gazing at the paper))
    C: ((putting her hand on T's shoulder))
    T: ((pushes her hand away while rocking))
    C: Look. (0.5) What did w[e forget?]
                             [(C points to ear piece on the paper)]
→   T: What did we: forge:t? The Nose. hh  ehn.
       ((stops rocking, picks up the other piece and starts gluing))
   C: okay.
   T: (20.0)((notetaking))
   T: ((puts the nose on the paper))
      (2.0)
   C: [Wha:::t else] is left.
      [(faces toward T)]
      (1.0)
```

```
     C: What's left?
     T: ((starts rocking))
     T: The ey::e.  An- h. (1.5)
        [(stops rocking and picks up one of the ear pieces,
        putting this on the paper)]
  →  T: [What's so- so- a:lso you left.]
        [(touching both ear pieces)]
     T: [The Ear.]
        [(picking up and start gluing and putting it on the table)]
     C: Right.
     T: (6.0)((continues gluing))
     C: [Put them on.]
     T: [(gluing)]
     C: [That's enough.]
     T: [(gluing and looking inattentively)]
     C: ((putting her hand on T's shoulder without actually touching))
     C: [Put it down. (2.0)You can stop now.]
        [(tapping on the table rightly) ]
        (10.0)
     C: We:: are all done.
        (2.0)
     C: Nice job.
```

Initially, the clinician complimented the child as he glued the required pieces onto the base paper (lines 1–5). Tony put his hand down on line 9 and directs his gaze toward the camera with a slight smile which could be suggestive of his task completion. On line 11, the clinician asked a question—"Are you all done?"—and immediately followed the question by informing Tony that they (i.e., Tony & Clinician) had forgotten one piece. This announcement can also function as directive as its action (cf. Schegloff, 2007: 9). At line 13, the clinician reformulated the question to produce a modally prefaced directive, "Can you find what we forgot?" suggestive (with the use of "we") of inclusive fault, but then later proposed Tony as the main agent responsible for the missing piece by saying "You forgot one thing" (line 15).

At lines 17 and 19, the clinician once again shifted the subject to "we," adding a more inclusive tone in directing. During these utterances, at line 18, the Tony began to exhibit some signs of distress (i.e., rocking on his chair). Furthermore, the clinician assisted with the task by pushing the correct piece toward the child, physically suggesting that he use the piece in the puzzle (lines 20–21). At line 25, the clinician re-issued the question—"What did we forget?" She prefaced this question with the word "look," which Sidnell (2007) shows is a canonical device for relaunching a course of action (in this case directing Tony toward the completion of the puzzle).

After these physical attempts (lines 20–26) toward guiding Tony, which he partially rejected by pushing away the clinician's hand, the Tony repeated the same directive at line 27.

Here is one focal utterance for our analysis. At line 27, Tony issued an echolalic repetition of the clinician's question and directly followed this with the answer (or the second part of the question–answer pair) by saying "the nose." The clinician acknowledged this answer in line 29 by saying "okay," while also making a note. Then, the child picked up the nose piece and began to apply glue and put the nose on the base (line 31).

After gluing the nose, the clinician asked, "wha:::t else is left?" (line 33), and then repeated the question on line 36. Tony answered with "the eye" in line 38. In another focal part of this episode, Tony mumbled slightly, and then repeated the clinician's question from line 33 at line 41, and answered it himself on line 43, saying "the ear." The clinician acknowledged this response (line 45), encouraged Tony (lines 47, 49), and proposed concluding the subtest on lines 51–57. Finally, she ended the exchange by way of a compliment, "NICE JOB" (line 57).

This use of echolalia immediately followed by the correct answer indicates the emergence of both components of an adjacency pair (Sacks et al., 1974), which are ordinarily produced by different parties to an interaction. The child's self-completion of these pair components is usually treated as an indication of the "loneliness of the autistic child" (Frith, 1989)—that is, the child's sense of confinement within the self. If the present case of echolalia is examined independently from the stream of interaction, it would indeed appear as being a product of the child's self-involvement. However, when considering it in the context of the entire interaction, it may reflect other features. First, the echolalia (lines 27, 41) appears to be a way for the child to delay answering while still introducing a relevant component of the talk—possibly processing the question in a way that projects an answer. Second, it can indicate that the child is exhibiting co-orientation with the clinician—as an aspect of the interactional substrate—and is following what the clinician is directing him to do.

Marking Bodily Alignment with Echolalia

A major part of co-orientation during testing episodes is how both the clinician and child position their bodies relative to one another and the tasks in which they are engaged (Maynard & Marlaire, 1992). For example, children may display recipiency toward a testing task by sitting in such a way that indicates that they are clearly prepared to engage in that task. In contrast, a child's rocking back and forth on his or her chair, or momentarily leaving the chair, may indicate the lack of co-orientation and readiness for a test item. Echolalia may occur at a point when the child represses the bodily rocking and shows greater recipiency.

Fragment 2 provides evidence of how echolalia shows interactional attentiveness. Note that Tony appeared to be inattentive or unaligned with the task orientation (lines 8 to 18), as evidenced by his rocking and appearing disengaged, until the point that he produced echolalia and a verbal answer to the question "What did we forget?" (lines 19–30). During this, the clinician called for his attention by placing her hand on his shoulder (line 23), which he rebuffed by pushing her hand away and continuing to rock (line 24). When Tony issued the repeated question and an answer (line 27), he stopped rocking (line 28) and began gluing the missing nose piece (line 31). In short, the echolalia was situated at the point where the rocking stopped (line 28) and engagement in—indeed, control over—the task began. This relationship between the cessation of rocking and verbal alignment was evident in the second instance of echolalia as well (lines 39–42). We address the import of this relationship between rocking and vocalizing below.

Multiple Productions of Echolalia Across Question–Answer Sequences

When an echolalic statement is repeated a number of times as part of the question–answer testing sequence, each instance may have different functions within the series of turns. In this case, multiple productions of echolalia invite further instructions.

Fragment 3 shows an example of repeated echolalia. This fragment occurs when the child was about to finish the little boy puzzle by gluing all the pieces. Following the clinician's question about where the child should put his name (line 12), the arrowed lines in the fragment indicate three productions of echolalia. The first instance (line 18) is repeated (23) and then partially repeated later (29).

Fragment 3

```
     C: Okay, Hey, I've got. some questions for you. Are you all
        done?
     T: Yaah. ((looking at the puzzle paper))
     C: That's very nice. Can [you put your name on there? (2.0)
                              [(putting the pencil in front of T)]
     T:  ((picking up the pencil and playing with it))
     C:  You write your name on there for me.
          (1.0)
     C:  You know how to write your name?
         (1.5)
     T: ((slowly holding the pencil in a writing style and facing
           toward the paper))
     C: Where (0.2) should you. You- where can you write your na:me.
     T: ((holding the pencil and shaking head tremblingly))

     T: [Enh. Enh.]
        [(looking at Clinician's face)]
     C: Can you?
 →   T: Where [ do you write your name?]
              [(continues looking at Clinician's face)]
     C: Where-? you, let's do it right he[re.
                                         [(pointing at the
        corner of the paper)]
 →   T: =Enh. Enh. (let's) should-  [let's shu- write
        your name?]
                                    [(looking up & lifting up
        shoulders)]
     C: Write it right [here.
                       [(pointing to the same place again)]
 →   T: Let's should, let's you (whe-  what's)
        your name?
        ((starts putting the pencil down on paper, looking
        at Clinician's face))
     C: (uhnn?) ((notetaking))
     T: ((starts writing)) ((rocking)) ((puts down the pencil))
        ((rocking))
     C:  Write the rest of it?
     T: ((stop rockings, picks up the pencil and start writing))
     C: Should we take it off so it doesn't break? ((paper sound)) Now,
        try.
        ((moving the board under the paper))
     T: ((stops writing, moving backward))
        ((starts writing))
        ((writing))
        ((puts the pencil down and picks up the
        paper))
        ((brings the paper to the Clinician))
     C: Hey, what does it say?
```

The echolalic utterances transpired as follows. First, the clinician initiated this segment by announcing the forthcoming testing task with "I've got some questions for you." She inquired about the completion of the puzzle (lines 1–2), which the child answered in the affirmative ("Yeah" on line 3). This completed a question–answer adjacency pair. The clinician subsequently provided a positive evaluation (line 4), thus completing a three-part testing sequence. Within the same turn as the evaluation, the clinician initiated the next testing sequence by asking whether the child can write his name on the finished puzzle (4), which is a kind of "directive" to do the task that encodes a degree of entitlement (Curl & Drew, 2008). However, this question was met with silence (end of line 4). Then, the clinician produced a more entitled directive ("You write your name ...," line 7), using imperative grammar. However, after another silence (line 8), the clinician asked whether Tony knew "how to write" his name, clearly orienting to the issue of his ability to do the task. Next, as Tony appeared ready to answer (lines 11–12), the clinician asked *where* Tony can write his name, suggesting her assessment that he could do it but needed to figure out the location for writing it.

As the clinician repeats her directive partially at line 17 by reverting to the "can you?" formulation, Tony responded to the statement with an echolalic repeating of the clinician's question using the *where* preface (line 18), rather than the "can you" uttered in the prior turn by the clinician. This suggests that Tony was claiming competence for writing his name (he "can") and, instead, that he might have been orienting to an issue of the location for his signature.

The first echolalia elicited an answer in the form of a clear instruction from the clinician of "Let's do it right there." Thus, the echolalia functioned here to obtain a concrete directional instruction utterance from the clinician. Similarly, the child's second repetition of the question (line 23) preserved an orientation to "where," and elicits a repetition of the location (line 26) using the imperative ("write it right here") rather than the inclusive ("let's do it ...," line 20). These first and second echolalic utterances, therefore, appear similar to the first type of echolalia shown in Fragment 1, in that they elicit responses from the clinician that suggest an orientation to Tony's indications of what sort of direction he needs.

The third instance of echolalia (line 29) did not receive a response from the clinician except for a small token (line 30) indicating simple recognition. In this third instance, Tony began writing immediately, and the clinician might have withheld verbal recognition as the indicated task was already in the process of being completed.

Echolalia in Suggestion–Agreement Sequences

When echolalia repeats a directive within a directive-response sequence, it may subsequently invite an "agreement" preferred by the initial suggestion (Pomerantz, 1984). In Fragment 4, Tony and the clinician have shifted to a different testing battery, requiring them to clear the pieces of a puzzle on which they had previously been working. The puzzle, which is a picture of a cow, is not yet completed. Tony has put the square puzzle pieces together into a rectangle without correctly ordering them.

Fragment 4

```
     C: Did you make a co::w? (1.5) Or you need a help?
     T:  ((turning around))
     T: I don't [need a help.
                [(looking away from the puzzle)]
     C: You do:n't. [Oka:y. (0.5)
     T:             [(facing toward the puzzle)]
     C: Okay, here,[you  know what?]
     T:            [(looking at her)]
     C: We got another puzzle here to make.(0.5) We gonna- do our own
        puzzle here.
     T: (1.0) ((touches the puzzle without moving pieces and continues
        touching the puzzle))
     C: Let's- let's put the cow away. We're all done with the
        cow.
  →  T: We are all done with the co::w.
     C: Yeah. Let's put the co:w away.
     T: (0.5)((picking up the puzzle)]
     C: ((placing hands on the table ))
     T: (2.5)((placing the puzzle on the clinician's hands while picking
        up more pieces))
     C: Thank you.
     T: (5.0)((changing the direction of pieces on the pile/putting them
        on her hand))
     C: Okay.
        ((taking the puzzle away))
```

After Tony strongly resisted having the clinician help him continue piecing together the cow (line 3), the clinician suggested moving on to the next puzzle (lines 7, 9–10). Tony continued to touch the puzzle pieces, seemingly "smoothing" the edges to create a straight rectangle out of the puzzle (lines 11–12). This suggests that he was not in alignment with the clinician's suggestion of starting the new puzzle. The clinician further directed Tony to "put the cow away" (line 13), announcing that they are "all done" (lines 13–14). Tony then repeated this utterance (line 15), which is received with an affirmative by the clinician, and an utterance directing the child to put the cow puzzle away (line 16). Thus, the echolalia here aligned to the clinician's trajectory, which he also followed with embodied activities—helping to pick up the puzzle pieces and putting them in the clinician's hands (lines 17–23).

Note that there is a similarity between this instance of echolalia and that described above, in relation to Fragment 1 (i.e., repetition of the question). This similarity can be summarized as follows:

Fragment 1

```
Clinician Question: Is that the way the pants go?
Tony Echo: Is that the way the pants go?
Clinician Confirm/Disconfirm: No.
Clinician Directive: You put them the way they go.
Tony Compliance: ((Turns the pants piece around))
```

Fragment 5

```
Clinician Directive: We're all done with the cow.
Tony Echo: We are ALL done with the cow.
Clinician Confirm/Disconfirm: Yeah.
Clinician Directive: Let's put the co:w away.
Tony Compliance: ((Picks up the cow pieces))
```

Both the question type and suggestion type of echolalia appear to facilitate achievement of the task at hand. More specifically, the locally produced task is carried out through the force of echolalia within a test sequence.

Conclusion

Close examination of immediate echolalia in a clinic for developmental disabilities revealed some of the ways in which this phenomenon is socially organized. By expanding the standard testing sequence (i.e., question-answer-evaluation), echolalia, as a facet of the interactional substrate, is a form of "concrete competence" (Maynard & Turowetz, 2017) that can enhance a child's performance. Our fragments show how Tony was able to solicit help from the clinician or complete the tasks in a self-regulatory manner. In addition, echolalia can expand the ordinary testing sequence in a way that allows for the exchange of more situated interactional cues, such as instructional utterances and confirming responses. Finally, as shown in Fragment 2, echolalia appeared at the point where the child stopped rocking. If the rocking indicated a need for coherence that was not being achieved verbally (Grinker, 2007: 186), it ceases at the moment when Tony showed himself—through the echolalia—to achieve such coherence by both *asking* and then *answering* the testing question. In short, a device in speech that traditionally has been seen as a deficit does not actually hinder, but rather enhances, the capacity of the child to perform particular tasks during testing. Through echolalia, children with Autism Spectrum Disorder are capable of producing relevant parts of the interactional sequences and adjust to requirements of the institutional setting.

The child with Autism Spectrum Disorder showed clear competency in this study which might disrupt preconceptions of these children's interactional disability. Indeed, close examination of this speech form, traditionally considered as deficit, can help us recognize how competent these children are in deploying the form as an interactional practice within a highly structured institutionalized setting. Often, people with recognizable disabilities are regarded as deviant and treated "not quite as humans"; they may be reduced from a whole person to a tainted, discounted, or stigmatized one (Goffman, 1963). This similarly applies to children with mental challenges, since their speech forms be taken as obvious or transparent indications of their disability. However, this study suggests that a particular speech form does not actually hinder, but rather enhances, the interactional accomplishment of testing tasks in institutionalized interactions.

The echolalia observed in this study reveals the numerous skilful interactional cues that facilitate a child with Autism Spectrum Disorder to achieve institutional tasks. When it involves repetition of a question or suggestion, echolalia avoids the sequential constraints of the moment, effectively shifting the conversational constraints to the other party. It also marks a point where the child is bodily aligned with a directive utterance placing a social constraint on him or her. When co-orientation is established, both bodily and verbally, echolalia can be used to initiate a child-owned conversational sequence. Following the echolalia, instructional utterances are produced and an interactional space is made, which may include extra conversational items. This permits the child to formulate his or her own interaction in a manner to which he or she is accustomed. The more the child creates a comfortable environment within which he or she can communicate in a routine way (e.g., using echolalia), the better he or she is able to adapt to changes in the situation.

Professional Reflection

Tetsuya Abe

Abstract

The empirical chapter on "Echolalia in clinical interaction" provides fine examinations of immediate echolalia during testing environment between a child with autism and a clinician. Echolalia is one of the popular symptoms in autism and has been understood as a neurological problem in developmental stage. In this reflection, I introduce three contributions this paper can offer to the medical field. First, autism has more social and interactional importance even though it is considered to have biological dysfunction in medical literature. Second, echolalia's communicative function has been recognized through a coding system. This paper shows richer description of its interactional function because of the sequential analysis of interaction. Third, proper responses towards echolalic utterances are useful to improve their communicative patterns. Conversation analysis can offer actual and practical examples of such interactionally appropriate responses.

This chapter provides fine-grained examinations of verbal and nonverbal aspects of immediate echolalia in a testing environment with a child with Autism Spectrum Disorder and a clinician. In this reflection, I would like to discuss three major contributions of this chapter for clinical practice.

First, this paper highlights the social and interactional importance in our conceptualization of Autism Spectrum Disorder. Autism Spectrum Disorder has been historically conceived as a behavioral disorder, characterized by lack of responsiveness toward others, noticeable developmental language disability, difficulties of building relationships with others, and a strong obsession toward repetitiveness. Recently, the DSM-5 (American Psychiatric Association, 2013) re-defines what is now known as Autism Spectrum Disorder, characterizing conditions along this spectrum as neurodevelopmental disorders that are manifested in communicational/social difficulties and local/repetitive behavioral patterns. This new category includes what has been previously defined as Autism Spectrum Disorder, Asperger's syndrome, and Pervasive Developmental Disorder.

Echolalia has been understood as a developmental neurological problem in the medical field. In typical development, children learn language through repetition. In the repetitive process, they usually learn to recognize the intention embedded within the repetitive utterances during an interaction. However, children with Autism Spectrum Disorder are believed to have a neurological disjuncture which presupposes the connection between automatic repetition and one's intention. Belmonte et al. (2004) explain this as abnormal neural connectivity, which can be found in their brain activity patterns. In the most of medical literature, echolalia has been considered to be solely a biological phenomenon. Thus, this paper can surely shed light on our understanding of echolalia by expanding our sociological and interactional understandings of this phenomenon.

Second, prior studies of echolalia have also recognized its communicative function (Prizant & Duchan, 1981). Prizant and Duchan (1981) developed a classical coding system of echolalia according to three aspects and displayed comprehension level, orientation toward interlocutors such as gaze and co-occurrence of physical behavior. Based on this coding scheme, they found seven functions of echolalia: non-focused, turn-taking, declarative, rehearsal, self-regulatory, yes-answer, and request. Most of all, their workplaces emphasis on the communicative function of echolalia. In the field of developmental education, their work has been cited as a major resource to understand echolalia as being functional instead of merely an abnormal form of speech. Nevertheless, although this research examined both verbal and nonverbal aspects of echolalia, it was limited to categorizing echolalia into the three above-mentioned characteristics. In the work of Prizant and Duchan (1981), however, the method of analyzing non-verbal aspects has not been fully developed. This limitation also has to do with its primary focus on individual capacity instead of understanding echolalia as being a more social and interactional phenomenon.

In addition, another previous study has examined what happens *before* the echolalic utterance. Rydell and Mirenda (1994) have focused on the nature of previous utterances, which occur before the echolalic utterance. They categorize the previous utterance into two groups: high and low constraint utterances. The high constraint utterances forced children to change their responses and behaviors such as directives whereas the low constraint utterances do not require the children to make such changes. As a result, echolalic utterances occur more often after the high constraint utterances.

On the contrary, this paper has offered its analysis based on more sequential organization of verbal behaviors based on conversation analysis, which allows us to acknowledge systematic details of the interaction. In Fragment 1, during the utterance of echolalia, the child is turning the puzzle toward right direction following the clinician's question "Is that the way the pants go?" Thus, this utterance shows understanding of the previous utterance. However, since the child is not looking at the clinician during this utterance, this utterance sounds more like self-talk. Thus, it can be considered as the type of echolalia called "self-regulatory" according to Prizant and Duchan (1981).

Furthermore, this paper includes analysis of what happens *after* the echolalic utterance. Thus, the analysis clarifies more functions of echolalia. First, with the echolalic utterance, the child can avoid social force posed by the clinician's question. Second, after the echolalic utterance, the clinician ends up assisting the child to complete the task at hand. Third, the child then accepts what the clinician did for him after the echolalic utterance. This paper has offered richer description of echolalia's interactional function because of its sequential analysis of interaction.

Third, this paper has the possibility of being applied to the interventions focused on the speech patterns of children with Autism Spectrum Disorder. There are many interventions that have been found to improve the particular speech patterns of children with Autism Spectrum Disorder (Hetzroni & Tannous, 2004; Lim & Draper, 2011; Matson, Sevin, Box, Francis, & Sevin, 1993). For example, Kurai (1997) reported on the importance of visual aids for instructing such children. When these children are asked questions along with visual aids such as pictures, it is easier for them to understand audio information of the question and to respond to the questions itself. These studies show the possibility of improving their communicational patterns by responding to echolalic utterances properly. However, it is quite difficult to determine what the "proper" responses can be toward echolalic utterances. Therefore, this kind of detailed analysis of interaction among children with Autism Spectrum Disorder and clinicians at institutional setting shown in this paper has its value because it can offer actual and practical examples of interactionally appropriate responses toward echolalic utterances.

References

American Psychiatric Association. (2013). *Diagnostic and statistical manual of mental disorders* (5th ed.). Arlington, VA: American Psychiatric Publishing.

Belmonte, M. K., Allen, G., Beckel-Mitchener, A., Boulanger, L. M., Carper, R. A., & Webb, S. J. (2004). Autism Spectrum Disorder and abnormal development of brain connectivity. *The Journal of Neuroscience, 20,* 9228–9231.

Clayman, S. E., & Gill, V. T. (2012). Conversation analysis. In J. P. Gee & M. Handford (Eds.), *The Routledge handbook of discourse analysis* (pp. 120–134). New York: Routledge.

Curl, T. S., & Drew, P. (2008). Contingency and action: A comparison of two forms of requesting. *Research on Language and Social Interaction, 41,* 129–153.

Fay, W. H. (1969). On the basis of autistic echolalia. *Journal of Communication Disorders, 2,* 38–47.

Frith, U. (1989). A new look at language and communication in autism. *International Journal of Language and Communication Disorders, 24*(2), 123–150.

Goffman, E. (1963). *Behavior in public places: Notes on the social organization of gathering.* New York: Free Press.
Gray, D. E. (2002) 'Everybody just freezes. Everybody is just embarrassed': Felt and enacted stigma among parents of children with high functioning Autism Spectrum Disorder. *Sociology of Health & Illness, 24*(6), 734–749.
Grinker, R. R. (2007). *Unstrange minds: Remapping the world of Autism Spectrum Disorder.* New York: Basic Books.
Heritage, J. (2005). Conversation analysis and institutional talk. In R. Sanders & K. Fitch (Eds.), *Handbook of language and social interaction* (pp. 103–147). Mahwah, NJ: Erlbaum.
Hetzroni, O. E., & Tannous, J. (2004). Effects of a computer-based intervention program on the communicative functions of children with Autism Spectrum Disorder. *Journal of Autism Spectrum Disorder and Developmental Disorder., 34*(2), 95–113.
Kurai, N. (1997). Jiheicyouna kodomo no shitumon-outou kannkei kunren (Training of question-response relationship for children with Autism Spectrum Disorder) *Gengo hattatsu chien kenkyu* (Studies on Retarded Language Development), *3*, 83–90 (in Japanese).
Lim, H. A., & Draper, E. (2011). The effects of music therapy incorporated with applied behavior analysis verbal behavior approach for children with Autism Spectrum Disorders. *Journal of Music Therapy, 48*(4), 532–550.
Marlaire, C., & Maynard, D. (1990). Standardized testing as an interactional phenomenon. *Sociology of Education, 63*, 83–101.
Matson, J. L., Sevin, J. A., Box, M. L., Francis, K. L., & Sevin, B. M. (1993). An evaluation of two methods for increasing self-initiated verbalizations in autistic children. *Journal of Applied Behavior Analysis, 26* (3), 389–398.
Maynard, D., & Marlaire, C. (1992). Good reasons for bad testing performance: The interactional substrate of education exams. *Qualitative Sociology, 15*(2), 177–202.
Maynard, D., & Turowetz, J. (2017). Doing testing: How concrete competence can facilitate or inhibit performances of children with Autism Spectrum Disorder. *Qualitative Sociology, 40*(4), 467–491.
Maynard, D., & Turowetz, J. (2019). Doing abstraction: Autism, diagnosis, and social theory. *Sociological Theory, 37*(1), 89–116.
Mehan, H. (1985). The structure of classroom discourse. In T. A. Dijik (Ed.), *Handbook of discourse analysis* (Vol. 3, pp. 120–131). New York: Academic Press.
Pomerantz, A. (1984). Agreeing and disagreeing with assessments: Some features of preferred/dispreferred turn shapes. In J. M. Atkinson & J. Heritage (Eds.),

Structure of social action: Studies in conversation. Cambridge: Cambridge University Press.
Prizant, B. M. (1978). *An analysis of the functions of immediate echolalia in autistic children* (Unpublished doctoral dissertation). State University of New York, Buffalo, NY.
Prizant, B. M., & Duchan, J. F. (1981). The functions of immediate echolalia in autistic children. *Journal of Speech and Hearing Disorder, 46*(3), 241–249.
Rydell, P. J., & Mirenda, P. (1994). Effects of high and low constraint utterances on the production of immediate and delayed echolalia in young children with Autism Spectrum Disorder. *Journal of Autism Spectrum Disorder and Developmental Disorder, 24*(6), 719–735.
Sacks, H. (1989). Lecture one: Rules of conversational sequence. *Human Studies, 12,* 217–227.
Sacks, H., Schegloff, E., & Jefferson, G. (1974). A simplest systematics for the organization of turn-taking for conversation. *Language, 50,* 696–735.
Schegloff, E. A. (1987). Analyzing single episodes of interaction: An exercise in conversation analysis. *Social Psychology Quarterly, 50*(2), 101–114.
Schegloff, E. A. (2007). *Sequence organization in interaction: A primer in conversation analysis, Volume 1.* Cambridge: Cambridge University Press.
Schuler, A., & Prizant, B. (1985). Echolalia. In E. Schopler & G. Mesibov (Eds.), *Communication problems in Autism Spectrum Disorder.* New York: Plenum Press.
Shapiro, T. (1977). The quest for a linguistic model to study the speech of autistic children. *Journal of the American Academy of Psychiatry, 16,* 608–619.
Sidnell, J. (2007). 'Look'-prefaced turns in first and second position: Launching, interceding and redirection action. *Discourse Studies, 9,* 387–408.
Sidnell, J., & Stivers, T. (2013). *Handbook of conversation analysis.* Boston, MA: Wiley-Blackwell.
Sterponi, L., & Shankey, J. (2014). Rethinking echolalia: Repetition as interactional resource in the communication of a child with Autism Spectrum Disorder. *Journal of Child Language, 41*(2), 275–304.
Tarplee, C., & Barrow, E. (2009). Delayed echoing as an interactional resource: A case study of a three year old child on the autistic spectrum. *Clinical Linguistics & Phonetics, 13*(6), 449–482.
Turowetz, J., & Maynard, D. W. (2017). Narrative methods for differential diagnosis in a case of Autism Spectrum Disorder. *Symbolic Interaction, 41*(3), 357–383.
Wootton, A. J. (1999). An investigation of delayed echoing in a child with Autism Spectrum Disorder. *First Language, 19,* 359–381.

4

Initiating Earthquake Talk with Young Children: Children's Social Competence and the Use of Resources

Amanda Bateman and Susan J. Danby

Professional Reflection by Paula Robinson and Claire Lethaby

Introduction

The importance of children receiving timely support to talk about past traumatic events is well-known in psychological research, where the process is intended to prevent the possibility of post-traumatic stress developing (National Institute of Clinical Excellence [NICE], 2005). In relation to the natural earthquake disaster in Christchurch New Zealand (February 2011), one such recovery strategy is 'Respond, Renew Recover', where

A. Bateman (✉)
Swansea University, Swansea, UK
e-mail: a.j.bateman@swansea.ac.uk

J. Lamerichs et al. (eds.), *Children and Mental Health Talk*,
The Language of Mental Health,
https://doi.org/10.1007/978-3-030-28426-8_4

the 'Recover' phase involves talking and recalling experiences in order to come to terms with the event (Brown, 2012). This chapter reveals how talk about the traumatic experiences of being involved in the Christchurch earthquake is initiated and managed in one early childhood centre through the everyday interactions between the teachers and children. We discuss the educators' use of supporting educational resources that respect the children's social competence in attending to their use and the social context to initiate conversations about the earthquake. The resources include Learning Story books, outdoor excursions to broken environments, and play equipment such as traffic cones and hard hats. The usefulness of these resources to initiate conversations that support recovery talk is demonstrated in transcriptions of unfolding talk about aspects of the earthquake event. The chapter includes a reflection by the teachers who were involved in the research. Their discussion reflects on the inclusion of these resources and their usefulness for initiating earthquake talk. Together, this chapter and the subsequent teacher reflection prompt other teachers to include such resources to help support children's recovery from traumatic experiences.

Context of the Project

On 22 February 2011 at 12.51 p.m., a 6.3 magnitude earthquake with a depth of only 5 km struck Christchurch, New Zealand Aotearoa. It resulted in the deaths of 185 people (NZ Police, 2012). One area of Christchurch that was particularly affected was New Brighton, where many buildings were severely damaged. As the earthquake occurred during the day, many people were at work and young children were at preschool.

S. J. Danby
School of Early Childhood and Inclusive Education, Queensland University of Technology, Brisbane, QLD, Australia
e-mail: s.danby@qut.edu.au

For the New Brighton Preschool, the earthquake came at the time of day when kai (meal) time had just finished and the youngest nursery children were asleep in their sleep room. When the earthquake struck, the quick-thinking actions of the early childhood teachers were paramount in ensuring the safety of all children present. The teachers gathered the young children who were awake onto the patch of grass in an open space in the preschool back garden so that they were out of reach of possible falling items that may have been loosened by the earthquake. The teachers gathered around the children in a protective circle in this outdoor space. Inside the building a similar protection of children was quickly initiated. Older children were encouraged to go under tables, with teachers following them so that they were on the outside, protecting the children from anything that might have fallen. Once the earthquake subsided, the older children who had been inside under the tables were taken outside to the grassy area so that they were with friends, but the toddler children were trapped inside the nursery. The teachers worked to gain access to the nursery to help the crying toddlers out of the earthquake-damaged room and eventually managed to open the stuck door to free them. Further actions to secure children's safety and well-being were managed as the teachers organized food, water, blankets and beanbags on the grass for all the children, as anxious parents began to arrive to collect their children. Throughout this traumatic experience, the teachers' actions demonstrated a provision of care for the children, as they grew increasingly aware of the possibility that some parents may have been severely affected by the earthquake and may possibly not arrive to pick up their child.

In the days and weeks that followed, an official response to managing the earthquake disaster unfolded. One initiative that was found particularly useful for those affected was the '3 Rs' (Respond, Recover and Renew) (Brown, 2012: 88). The 'Recover' aspect of this 3-phase response highlighted the importance of talking about experiences in order to allow 'emotional recovery' and progress in making sense of events. Particular connections were made to the New Zealand early childhood curriculum *Te Whāriki* (Ministry of Education [MoE], 1996/2017), where there is an holistic approach to education, and explicit mention of supporting children's 'emotional well-being' (pp. 15, 46 and 50), 'emotional robustness' (p. 21) and 'emotional security' (p. 22). The curriculum is foregrounded in sociocultural theory where children are perceived as socially competent members of society who have strengths and funds of knowledge that they contribute to society. *Te Whāriki* is founded on the following aspirations for children:

> to grow up as competent and confident learners and communicators, healthy in mind, body, and spirit, secure in their sense of belonging and in the knowledge that they make a valued contribution to society. (MoE, 1996: 9)

The vision of children as active agents in everyday interaction encourages early childhood teachers to value the contributions of infants, toddlers and young children in everyday interactions so that they are supported to be 'competent, confident learners who ask questions and make discoveries' (MoE, 1996: 68). In understanding how conversations about the earthquake disaster are initiated in order to begin this process of recovery and renewal; this chapter focuses on how disclosures about the earthquake were initiated in situ with a focus on children's social competence in this co-construction.

Initiating Interactions

This chapter brings a sociological focus of inquiry to the everyday interactions that occurred between the teachers and the children, and among the children themselves, to show everyday scenes as they dealt with the trauma caused by the earthquake events. Bringing a situated perspective to the activity makes possible a focus on specific events through focusing on how the participants attend to the interactions occurring. In attending to the visible and audible structures of their talk-in-interaction, we show how the participants work at co-producing their social activities. The focus is not on children's words alone, nor their developmental capabilities, but rather how they engage with others (teachers, children) to make sense of their everyday worlds. This is particularly relevant when their everyday worlds were so disrupted by the extraordinary earthquake events.

Three fundamental assumptions underpin our understandings of social interaction (Heritage, 1984). First, social interaction is structurally organized. By this, we mean that there are stable patterns of talk that are organized in conversations, and we can study talk as social organization as a topic in its own right. For example, turn-taking is a structurally organized feature of talk. Second, the sequence of talk is important. Interactions are dependent upon preceding talk, and that talk forms the basis of what is said next. In other words, conversation is both context-shaped and context-renewing (Heritage, 1984). It is context-shaped because of a speaker's contribution in an ongoing sequence of talk, and it is context-renewing because the next speaker's turn is formed from the current speaker's immediate context. As well as talk, it is also important in face-to-face interactions to know what gestures (e.g. pointing) and other non-verbal actions (e.g. smiling) occur as these become a shared resource for participants. Within this framing, participants assemble possible meanings drawn from the situated context of the social interaction. These turns at talk are jointly produced by the members present and begin in orderly and structured ways (Sacks, 1992).

Elsewhere, we have described how children spontaneously re-enacted and talked about their trauma around the earthquake event through play (Bateman & Danby, 2013; Bateman, Danby, & Howard, 2013b; Bateman, Howard, & Danby, 2015). These experiences, self-initiated by the children, were serendipitous moments where the teachers initiated talk about the earthquake alongside the children's play activities. The teachers in our study interacted in ways with the children that produced talk that was similar to therapeutic interactions in a clinical setting. For example, therapists may join in with the child's play to provide opportunities to support the child to understand the event and, consequentially, to reframe the children's trauma responses (Prendiville, 2014). Other therapeutic strategies include creative arts-based activities such as drama and performance to create an emotional distance from the event to facilitate healing (O'Connor, 2012). Negative exposure therapy supports children to construct narratives of their experiences in order to become children to relive these experiences to become more habituated to those experiences of trauma (Ruf et al., 2010). Institutional helplines such as the Australian Kids Helpline offer a safe and caring environment where they support the young callers to communicate their troubles, and counsellors provide counselling support through promoting self-directed solutions (Danby, Butler, & Emmison, 2011). Although professional counsellors can offer essential healing, an approach involving non-specialist staff such as parents, teachers and friends also has been found to be effective in supporting children through traumatic events to begin the process of recovery and healing (Gibbs, Mutch, O'Connor, & MacDougall, 2013). This chapter now explores the initiation of earthquake talk between children and their teachers.

The Project

The imperative for the project was an exploration of how children and teachers were responding in their everyday interactions with each other in the days that followed the earthquake. The project catalyst was initiated by parents and early childhood teachers requesting knowledge about how to best support their children through recovery (Dean, 2012). The project aim was to reveal what was happening in everyday practices, so that lessons could be learnt regarding how earthquake talk was being managed in situ. To begin the project, ethical approval was gained from the University of Waikato Ethics Committee, followed by the Preschool Centre director, the parents of the children and, finally, the children. All families agreed to full consent for their children, and all children also agreed to take part, resulting in fifty-two child participants. All nine teachers consented to be involved in the study.

The principal investigator (Amanda Bateman) video recorded everyday interactions between children and teachers to see how the participants oriented to the earthquake in their everyday talk. Video recordings of children's everyday interactions provided unique access to the children's cultures, to which adults might not otherwise gain. Video footage affords researchers repeated access to the recorded interactions so that the interests of the participants can be viewed and transcribed in fine detail, allowing researchers opportunities to learn from the interactions viewed (Pink, 2013; Sacks, 1984).

A total of eight hours and twenty-one minutes of footage was collected over the duration of one week at the preschool. Video recordings captured moments when the earthquake was talked about and also play that included fixing broken things. These video recorded episodes were transcribed using conversation analysis transcription conventions (Jefferson, 2004) to reveal detailed features of talk, of what was said by whom in the sequence of the interaction, and also *how* it was said in order to reveal the social organization in interaction. Some context of the study of initiating conversations by making use of conversation analysis is now given.

Conversational openings were explored as a significant part of everyday interaction in the early work of conversation analysis (Sacks, Schegloff, & Jefferson, 1974; Schegloff, 1968). Initiations of such openings work to secure an interaction, as one person's first pair part (FPP) occasions a second pair part (SPP) from another person (Sacks et al., 1974). When a person initiates an interaction with someone through a FPP, they often will use a pre-sequence to ensure that they have the attention of the targeted person before progressing to continue with the interaction. Sacks (1992) suggests that a FPP involves the use of a pre-sequence in order to gauge how their utterance will be received. The recipient shows their willingness to contribute to the interaction through their response, which either can be verbally expressed or non-verbally implemented through actions such as gaze bodily alignment and facial expression (Goodwin, M. H., 2006; Goodwin, C., 2017).

The sequence of exchanges in opening an interaction is observable in everyday interactions, making everyday scenes visible. For example, a question goes before an answer, 'there is plainly, hearably, a first greeting and a greeting return; they're said differently' (Sacks, 1992: 521). Questions often are used as a way of securing an interaction with someone and are used especially by children (Sacks, 1992). Sacks (1992) also suggests that, in the opening of an interaction, people may refer to conversational tickets or objects that can be used as an account for why one person initiates contact with another. Conversational tickets are structured so that they orient to the reason why one person is approaching another, such as asking for the time or for directions (Sacks, 1992). This use of objects for initiating interaction has been explored in prior work (Bateman & Church, 2017) where four-year-old children were found to co-construct the order of the playground through orienting to environmental features and any available objects. In this chapter, we show how teachers and children initiate and organize their talk-in-interaction around environmental resources to accomplish shared meanings about events related to the earthquake and the consequences in their everyday lives post-earthquake.

Data and Analysis

Orientation to Environmental Resources for Initiating Earthquake Talk

The importance of being physically present in the earthquake-damaged environment was relevant for prompting discussion and reflection on the earthquake experiences. There were many buildings that had suffered various levels of damage around the preschool location, and these were unavoidable upon entering and exiting the preschool. We now show how the teachers and children oriented to some aspects of the earthquake-damaged environment and not to others.

Direct Initiation of Earthquake Recall

Fragment 1 shows how the teacher uses everyday sand play to prompt talk about liquefaction. The preschool teacher Lorraine (LOR) is sitting next to the sandpit where many of the children are playing. One preschool girl, Maiah (MIA), is sitting on her lap and 3 other girls (Chloe—CLO; Sienna—SNA; and Milika—MKA) are crowded around her. The teacher begins with some questions designed to prompt memories of the earthquake event and to prime the children in terms of thinking about their daily lives following the earthquakes.

Fragment 1 Bateman and Danby (2013)

LOR: does anybody remember when we had <liquefaction> in our
ro↑ads (1.4) and <u>sink</u> ho:les? (0.8) what did sink holes
do¿
(2.4)
BAX: they make- they make <<u>wa:ter</u>>↓
LOR: do they make wa:ter¿
(0.7) ((*children look at the sand*))
LOR: what sort of water¿.was it clear wa:ter or ↓muddy water.
what sort of water↓
CLO: clear water
LOR: clear water¿.and who had some big pot-holes in their
hou↓ses?
MKA: ((*raises her hand*))
LOR: you did Milika¿.what did- what can you tell me about
<your> house¿
CLO: ↑when the earthquake- when the earthquake- when the
earthquake ↓flooded ↑it all get flooded¿
LOR: it ↑did flood ↓did your house- did=you=your=house
have lots of flooding?
CLO: ye↑ah¿
LOR: it did?
(0.2)
LOR: and ↓do you know Alex said to me yesterday? he had tracks
down his hou- down- down his road¿
CLO: [yeah]
SNA: [mine] did too::
LOR: did you too↓
SNA: >yes< in my old broken house that got broked¿
LOR: what happened¿ did you have to move ↑out Sienna¿
SNA: ↓yea:h? Ruahine
LOR: you what?
SNA: Ru↑ahine¿
LOR: Ruahine
SNA: ((*nods head*))
LOR: what does Ruahine mean¿ (1.7) oh where you used to
live in Bexley¿
SNA: ((*nods head*))
LOR: and your house got all <u>broken</u>¿
SNA: °yeah°

Counselling guidelines often recommend the strategy of avoiding questions when discussing traumatic events with children, as counsellors are not familiar with the children's prior experiences (Graffam Walker, 2013). The preschool context shown here, however, is not a formal counselling context. Teachers, because of their daily interactions with children, often do have a substantial knowledge about children's lives, including knowledge about family members, where they live, and prior experiences as shared by the children and families. This shared knowledge is readily available and becomes a resource for the teacher, as shown in this particular sequence of talk.

This sequence of talk is triggered by the children's investigations of liquefaction in the sandpit, and the teacher uses this experimentation to initiate a sequence of questions about their memories. She begins by asking children to remember, first, about the sinkhole and, next, about the potholes. While she does not specifically refer to the earthquake, it is clear that the children make the connection to the earthquake in their subsequent talk, demonstrated by Chloe in her explicit mention (lines 16–17). The teacher's approach both prompts talk about a particular topic—liquefaction—and provides interactional space for the children to initiate explicit references to the earthquake if they chose to do so.

After Chloe produces her first telling prompted by the teacher's questions, and the teacher initiates a second telling recounting a conversation she had recently (lines 21–24). In introducing this topic, done as a retelling of a conversation with another child, she shapes this in a way so that others, including Sienna, also contribute their recalls to the collective group. When one story leads to another, these stories are described as 'second stories' (Sacks, 1992). A second story is designed to show mutual attention towards both the talked about event and associated understanding displays of 'recognizable similarity' (Arminen, 2004: 319). Here, we see that the telling offered also follows this systematic format. As well as clearly displaying association with the first telling and a shared experience, the teller identifies with the prior teller and their experiences, and as such reminds children that they are not alone in relation to their experiences of the earthquake. The teacher's use of questions about the environmental resources works to orient the children to the concept of liquefaction and to link that back to the earthquake event, which produces the context for the production of reflective recalls here. This orientation to environmental resources to prompt earthquake recall is also evident in the subsequent transcriptions and so appears to be a common practice in these teacher–child interactions.

On the Way to the Hole in the Road

Fragment 1 showed how a particular environmental feature was talked into importance by the teacher and children, and how the unfolding talk prompted a connection to the earthquake. The same type of strategy is used in the following interaction shown in Fragment 2.

This event occurred in the morning when children and teachers found that, on entering the early childhood centre, there was no water. After some investigation through talking about the situation with others, the teachers found that the earthquake had caused the tarmac of a nearby road to weaken. The road had given way when a large lorry had driven over it, causing damage to the underlying water pipe. As each experience like this was treated as a learning opportunity by the teachers, the children, Myla (MYL) and Sienna (SNA) and teacher Pauline (PLN) went to investigate the situation. The following sequence shows how the teacher initiates talk about the earthquake through an environmental noticing.

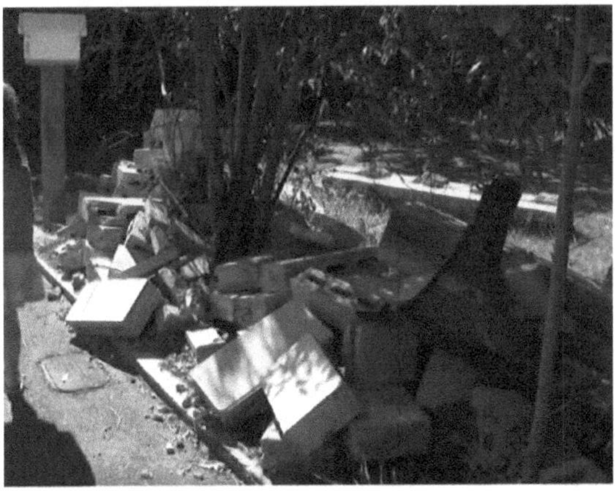

Fragment 2 (Bateman, Danby, & Howard, 2013a)

```
01 PLN:    Oh¿ ↑lo::ok?
02         (2.0)
03         what's tha:t. he:re?
04         ((looks at a broken breezeblock wall))
05 MYL:    Uh::?
06 PLN:    what¿- (1.4) I wonder what happened there?
07 MYL:    °↓ I dunno° ((looks at the wall and then
08         the teacher))
09 PLN:    ↑dunno?
10 SNA:    oh? there was something there?=
11 PLN:    =°↓something (     ) I wonder how [the-°?
12 MYL:                                      [I think-
13         I think it's from the ea::rthquake↓
```

At the beginning of this sequence, the teacher makes a noticing by drawing attention to the broken wall. She does so without giving additional information about what to 'look at' or why, accomplishing this initial noticing with gesture as well as her verbal opening as she looks at the wall. The teacher manages this initial opening by using a pre-sequence (line 1) to ensure that she has secured the attention of the children before progressing further with the interaction and specifically draws their attention to an environmental feature. There are various types of pre-sequences that are used to establish activities in the initiation of a preferred, agreeable interaction (Schegloff, 2007) where they are used as introductions to subsequent talk (Schegloff, 1980). Here, this pre-sequence solicits the attention of the children, while also initiating the progression of the interaction to be around the topic of the broken wall.

Following this first noticing 'oh look', there is a two-second silence where there was opportunity for the children to contribute; another common practice, but as there was no immediate response, Pauline continues with 'what's that here'. This utterance draws further attention to the broken wall, so that Pauline's initiation of this sequence consists of a double attention elicit involving the environmental feature in her conversational opener. This time, she uses a question in her FPP to make the response of an answer relevant. In doing so, she sets up a specific topic of talk from the beginning of the interaction in her FPP, prompting a specific type of SPP response from the children that will be obliged to be about the object she has attended to (Sacks, 1992). As with Fragment 1, the orientation to environmental resources is evident here in prompting children to engage in talk about the earthquake.

Pauline's initiation of this interaction uses a question that prompts the children to reply with a demonstration of their knowledge, acknowledging the children's competence and giving them the opportunity to contribute. Myla responds with a minimal response token (line 5), which requires Pauline to reformulate her question, again offering the children the opportunity for contribution. In Pauline's next turn at talk (line 6), she uses 'I wonder' to prompt a knowledge display from the recipients (Houen, Danby, Farrell, & Thorpe, 2016a, 2016b). Even though the next couple of lines (7–8) suggest a lack of engagement, another child then does attend to the wall (line 10), prompting Myla to then offer her contribution of knowledge (lines 12–13).

Through progressing with this enquiry as an opening of interaction in this focused way, Pauline acknowledges the children's competence by providing opportunity for them to offer their hypothesis around what has happened, even if they do not know the 'correct' answer. This opportunity is subsequently picked up by Myla who offers a hypothesis for why the wall is broken by orienting to the earthquake, demonstrating her knowledge and understanding of events. Myla's response to the initiated topic provides opportunity for Pauline to follow Myla's interest and understanding of events by unpacking further issues surrounding the earthquake. This sequence demonstrates how initiating an interaction through an environmental noticing by using 'I wonder' and leaving pauses has sequential opportunities for children to show their competence in talking about their earthquake experiences.

The Hole in the Road

Continuing from the walk-in Fragment 2, the children Myla (MYL), Sienna (SNA), Lucy (LCY), and Cayden (CDN), and teachers Pauline (PLN) and Sandra (SDR) finally reach the hole in the road, where more talk about the earthquake is prompted.

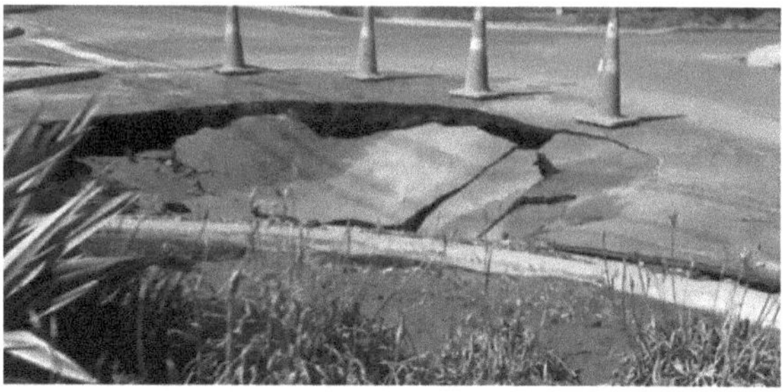

Fragment 3 (Bateman et al., 2013a)

71 PLN: come here have a look so you can see¿
72 (1.6) ((children position around the hole))
73 MYL: I can't see?
74 PLN: loo::k↓
75 (0.6) ((all looking at the hole in the road))
76 look at that ↓huge hole?
77 SDR: look what happened from the ↑earthquake.
78 PLN: it's part of the ↑road isn't it.
79 ?: yeah
80 (3.8) ((children re-position around the hole))
81 PLN: I think (1.4)
82 SNA: [(Myla can't go that way)]
83 PLN: [l a s t   n i g h t] the water pipes broke under
84 there and then the water came up and it
85 made the road break¿
86 MYL: what?
87 PLN: all the wa:ter: in the pipe- the pipes
88 broke¿
89 MYL: o↓h
90 PLN: they (0.5) got loose in the earthquake
91 (3.1) and then it all come flooding up and
92 it's broken the road¿
93 LCY: that was the truck we saw ((*points to a*
94 *passing vehicle*))
95 PLN: you can stay there (0.3) stay there.
96 ((*walks towards the edge of the hole*))
97 ((*3 children have a brief conversation*
98 *nearby*))
99 (19.2)
100 PLN: Cayden? (0.3) have they fixed all the road
101 in your street?
102 CDN: ((*looks at Pauline and nods head*))
103 PLN: was your hole as big as that?
104 CDN: ((*looks at the hole and then back at Pauline.*
105 *Shakes his head*)) My hole was deeper than that¿

As in Fragment 1, Pauline initiates the interaction by making a noticing about a specific environmental feature, prompting the children to come and look at it, placing emphasis on gaining visual access to *see* it (lines 71–76). This initial noticing is followed with a significant gap in the talk of over a second while the teacher shepherds the children (Cekaite, 2010) around the hole. This gap in the talk, although used to position children, also affords opportunity for the children to contribute their opinion and/or knowledge about the environmental feature; a common practice found in the data discussed in this chapter. Ending this gap with her response, Myla also orients to the need to *see* the environmental feature that Pauline is drawing her attention to, highlighting the need for first-hand knowledge of the scene. First-hand knowledge can be secured through being an eye-witness to an event, as physically observing specific episodes can provide authentic experience through connecting with emotions (Hutchby, 2001). Through providing an opportunity for the children to see the environment in post-earthquake state, the teachers provide legitimate first-hand knowledge for the children in a situation where they can ask questions and offer their knowledge about the event. As such, these experiences afford tools and knowledge to talk about events with children in the process of their recovery (Brown, 2012).

Pauline continues drawing the children's attention to 'look', repeating the word twice and with emphasis, and this time is more specific about which environmental feature to which she is directing their attention—'that huge hole'—in order to gain understanding. This prompt is followed by a second teacher, Sandra, also asking the children to 'look' (line 77). Sandra's guidance for the children to 'look' makes the first specific mention of the earthquake in this interaction, as she tells the children it is the reason for the road being broken (line 77). Pauline takes the opportunity to talk to the children about factual knowledge around the broken road here, and how it is related to the recent earthquake. Towards the end of this interaction (lines 100–105), Pauline prompts Cayden to contribute to this topic by acknowledging that he has knowledge that is worthy of sharing, demonstrating that his contribution is valued, and presenting him as competent in adding to the knowledge that is already being shared. Cayden does contribute, initially through gesture as he nods his head in response to Pauline's question, and then verbally where he offers news that the hole in his street is deeper than the one they are currently looking at, disclosing details about the impact of the earthquake.

The sequences reveal how an impromptu physical exploration of an environmental feature related to the recent earthquake can provide opportunity for spontaneous earthquake talk. The teacher initiated the topic by orienting to specific environmental features that she encouraged the children to engage with first-hand and offered facts about the earthquake and the damage it caused. As such, this sequence of verbal actions worked to provide an opportunity for the children to contribute their knowledge in competent ways, so to build a clearer understanding of the impact of the earthquake from equally valued various perspectives.

Learning Story Books: Important Documentation for Initiating Reflection

At the beginning of the research project, the children at the early childhood centre were informed that the researcher was interested in hearing their stories about the earthquake, and this introduction was enough to prompt some children to recall events without further prompting. The following three fragments reveal how Learning Story books, used to document children's learning and prompt reflection on that learning, are an important resource for recording children's earthquake experiences for later revisiting. The Learning Stories approach is a formative assessment for children attending early childhood education in New Zealand, where episodes of children's learning are documented for reflection, supporting children to see themselves as capable and confident learners (Carr & Lee, 2012). Teachers document the learning of each child by writing a story to the child about their learning accomplishments, where there is great focus on children's competence. Each child has their own collection of stories that are produced into books for the children to keep and reflect on throughout their continuous educational journey.

The following two fragments (4 and 5) show how two of the four-year-old children competently initiated an interaction with the researcher using their Learning Story books to tell about their earthquake experiences; Fragment 6 shows a collaborative remembering of the earthquake between a teacher and child using his Learning Story book.

Baxter and His Learning Stories

In Fragment 4, one child, Baxter (BAX), showed the researcher his book and started talking specifically about the earthquake events that he had documented in there. This was an extended turn at talk where the researcher did not say anything. Baxter talks and turns his pages simultaneously, where the pictures and words support his telling about his earthquake experience.

Fragment 4 (Bateman, Danby, & Howard, 2013b, 2016)

```
BAX:   so these two trucks he:re¿ ((points to
       page)) they broke coz coz w- coz w- coz tha- ther-
       some of them got broken coz coz from the
       earthquake s- so um w- we got some <ne:w> trucks and
       some steel loa:ders .hhh and (0.2) th- we still got these
       (0.2) rollers¿ ((points to picture)) and and
       then we h went to (turns page) have a look and
       .hhh and we saw this ((points to picture and moves
       finger in a circular motion)) big big digger and .hhh
       (1.1) then one day ((turns page)) from the
       ea:rthqu↑ake we- we- me and Corbin and my mum and my
       friend Sandra . and . Pete . and . (0.3) his other friend
       comed around and had a look but <we> had a first
       look .hhh so we- so we- um we did it all in .hhh
       here ((points to picture)) with (0.3) u- with my
       friend Corbin with somviva- survival jackets from
       my hou- .hhh some from from actually Sandra bought it
       that day ((turns page)) .hhh so then (0.8) Corbin
       didn't want it so I- so he took it off .hhh so then um
       they were maked a <ne:w> fence (0.6) ((looks at
       researcher and then out of the window and points
       towards the window)) of over there and (0.2) .hhh so
       tha:t's ((points to picture)) the same fence as that
       one ((points towards the window)) and then ↑this
       fence ((points to picture)) broked fr- from the
       <earth:>quake
((continues talking about events documented in his book))
```

Baxter is using one of his Learning Story books to tell stories about his earthquake experience to the researcher who is video recording him. Although the prior fragments demonstrated how a teacher's orientation to an environmental resource was used to prompt earthquake talk with the children, the prompt for earthquake talk here comes from the documentation in Baxter's Learning Story book. He competently offers a telling of news about events that he experienced first-hand, as documented in his book through writing and photographs of people, places and things. As with Fragments 1 and 2, his documented first-hand knowledge highlights the importance of being a present eye-witness (Hutchby, 2001). Baxter orients to this first-hand experience when he competently recalls a list of people who were physically present at the time, as he makes his disclosure about events, often using gesture as he points to specific pictures as he talks. In this particular part of the telling (lines 11–12), Baxter uses self-repair from 'we' to an actual list of names of the group, and photographs in his Learning Story book to stress the importance of being as accurate as possible when recalling this earthquake story, and so offers further validation of his story (Sacks, 1992). Baxter's recipient design in his telling can be observed, where he offers specific names of members to which the researcher would not otherwise have access. Baxter's subsequent orientation to having a 'first look' (lines 13–14) also demonstrates the importance placed on being present and being first with the news (Sacks, 1992).

Whereas the prior fragments demonstrated the usefulness of exploring damaged environments for initiating talk about earthquake experiences and offering opportunities for children to contribute their knowledge, here we see that Learning Story books can be equally as important resources for facilitating such talk. The way in which Baxter attends to each page in the process of telling his earthquake stories reveals the vital role that the documented stories and pictures played for such important disclosures when the stories were revisited. When reflecting on the story of the fence (lines 20–26), Baxter switched from past to present changing from 'that' (line 23) to 'this' (line 24) with emphasis placed on these words, while referring to the fence as a pivotal utterance to link his present situation with his past earthquake one (Bateman et al., 2013b). Learning Story books can be valuable artefacts for prompting and reflecting on earthquake experiences.

The observable way that Baxter used each page and picture to prompt his specific tellings (noted by the page turning) indicates the importance he placed on using Learning Story books to document events that can be returned to in the iterative process of coming to terms with an event (Brown, 2012). By documenting events in Learning Story books, the books provide a valuable resource for initiating talk and reflective thought, as also evident in the next transcription.

Cayden and His Learning Stories

Cayden (CDN) approached the researcher and asked if he could show her his book. The researcher accepted, and Cayden placed his book on the table and opened it on a page about the earthquake. Cayden held the clip-on microphone close to his mouth and began speaking into it while pointing, with his other hand, to the picture in his book.

Fragment 5 (Bateman et al., 2013b, 2016)

CDN: the- the ↑**ear**thquake breaked the stuff¿ so we-
so we didn't ↑go ↓there (0.3) .hhh coz
there was there was ↑lots of <ho:les> (0.5) .hhh and
and er ((*turns 2 pages*)) oopsy ((*looks at*
Baxter and turns 1 page back)) coz the
↑earthquake was <**st**ro:ng>¿ (0.4) .hhh and- and-
BAX: and it $**broke** our fe:nce$¿ ((*laughs and leans towards*
Cayden and makes eye contact))
CDN: and it broked . the preschool's . fence¿ ((*looks at his*
book))

As with Fragment 4, Cayden immediately begins talking about the earthquake as documented in his book and using the words and pictures about the earthquake as support. Cayden places emphasis on the earthquake breaking things and creating holes, which becomes significant when we see that in Fragment 2 Pauline asks Cayden about the hole in *his* road, indicating that Cayden has documented this experience and is now recalling it. The documentation in the Learning Story book, as well as excursions to the broken environment, provides different types of opportunities for initiating earthquake talk for reflecting on past events and coming to terms with events. What is significant here, and in Fragment 4, is the competent ways in which Baxter and Cayden use their books to articulate the earthquake experiences that are of significance to them.

Leonie and Zack Read Zack's Learning Story Book

In this interaction, the early childhood teacher, Leonie (LEO) and 3 children are sitting on the grass in the preschool outdoor area. Each child is looking at their own Learning Story book, when the book becomes the stimulus for recalling the events around the earthquake. Two children leave and Leonie and Zack (ZAC) remain. The following interaction occurs:

Fragment 6 (Bateman & Danby, 2013)

```
01 ZAC:   ↑now can you read ↓mi:ne:?
02 LEO:   ar=↑sure:↓ . and that was all about the ↓earthquake
03        wasn't it >remember=when=we< had the
04        <earthqu:ake::> can you remember about the
05        earth↑quake::?
06 ZAC:   ↑yeah↑=
07 LEO:    =what can you remember about the earth↑quake¿
08 ZAC:   [    ↑mmmm¿     ]                [we:: (         )]
09 LEO:   [wha:t special] thing could [↑you remember¿]
10 ZAC:   on the grass?
11 LEO:   we did did↑n't we::¿ . and we all [came on to-]
12 ZAC:                                     [↑I remember] we-
13        I remember- I remember it?
14 LEO:   ↑you rem↓ember it? ↓can you remember what happened?
15        (0.9)
16 ZAC:    °mmm the dinosaurs-° the ↑di:nosaurs were dancing¿
17 LEO:    the ↑dinosaurs were dancing¿
18         (0.7)
19 LEO:    ↑real:ly:¿
```

This interaction around the documented earthquake Learning Story in the Learning Story book has been analysed previously to reveal how remembering the earthquake was a collaborative matter—a process that helped make sense of what happened during a tumultuous event (Bateman & Danby, 2013). Here, we focus on how the topic of the earthquake was initiated through the presence of the Learning Story book resource, affording opportunity for Zack to knowledgeably and competently disclose his memory of the earthquake in a secure environment with his teacher. Here, the teacher uses Zack's Learning Story book to prompt earthquake talk, and also uses pauses and gaps in talk to afford Zack an opportunity to contribute, both common practices used by the teachers' interactions, as shown in this chapter.

As with Baxter and Cayden, Zack initiates the reading of his Learning Story book by independently turning the book to the page where the earthquake is documented. Rather than reading the selected story to an audience, however, Zack hands the book to his teacher Leonie and asks her if she can read it (line 1). In doing so, Zack competently communicates to his teacher that he would like the focus of the story sharing to be about the earthquake. Leonie notices the story topic and recognizes the initiation from Zack as an important moment, responding in a way that prompts Zack to recall his earthquake experience (lines 2–5). This sequence of notice, recognize and respond is practised by early childhood teachers in their everyday pedagogy in New Zealand to support and extend children's learning experiences (Carr & Lee, 2012). Here, the learning experience is centred around recalling the earthquake through the 'revisiting' process, affording the opportunity for recovery through the iterative process of recalling experiences in order to come to terms with events (Brown, 2012). Zack then embraces the opportunity to demonstrate his competence in offering a hypothesis about what happened during the earthquake (line 16), further demonstrating the importance of documenting events and revisiting them in Learning Story books.

Discussion and Conclusion

Trauma is profoundly unsettling and distressing, and children who have experienced such events are likely to receive specialist support in the form of counselling or therapy. This process often involves maximizing children's capacity to disclose and describe the traumatic event, develop new ways to deal with their emotions, and develop new perspectives of the event and of themselves (Bateman et al., 2015).

An investigation of how children and teachers invoke talk about their traumatic experiences requires detailed insights into the systematic ways in which they introduce and discuss their experiences of trauma. In the episodes discussed in this chapter, we see two main common practices that prompt earthquake talk from the children: (1) orientation to environmental resources and (2) pauses and gaps in conversation that afford the child the opportunity to contribute their earthquake experiences. The teachers' interactions with the children produced conversations that invoked memories of the earthquake for both teachers and children. These accounts often began with an account of a memory of what happened when the earthquake occurred in terms of how they responded to this traumatic event, and the damage sustained to the community. As shown in these examples, these reported memories also became the interactional resources to reshape their accounts of that eventful day and aftermath. These reshaped accounts shifted to more positive discussion of how the community is being repaired, how community members were helping each other, and alternative ways to describe the earthquake that were more playful (e.g. Fragment 6, 'the dinosaurs were dancing').

The strategy of recalling experiences of traumatic events is important in children's lives in the process of the strategy of Respond, Renew and Recover (Brown, 2012). As the analysis highlighted, walks with children and the children's Learning Stories books support the children's telling. Further, the teacher's use of questions was designed to prompt displays of remembering. Engaging with the immediate environment and Learning Story books worked as extra props for the teacher's work, affording the opportunity for the children to recount their experiences. The teacher's probing through questions was undertaken in a peer context and, when the children gave their accounts, the reported memory was undertaken within a social context. This multiparty talk was heard by those present, as each built on the other's account, providing opportunity for accumulative knowledge through collective accounts that build ways to normalize and further understand the experience for the children.

The study has potential limitations in that the participants were aware that the researcher was particularly interested in the earthquake. This aligns with prior conversation analysis work with young children (Ekberg, Danby, Houen, Davidson, & Thorpe, 2017), where it is possible that the researcher's topic of interest impacted on the frequency of discussion of that specific topic. However, similar to the Ekberg et al. (2017) study, much of the footage collected did not include any discussion of the earthquake, suggesting that the children's interests were the main focus of everyday discussion rather than the researcher's primary interests.

Understanding children's spontaneous talk with their peers and teachers about their earthquake experiences, and the teachers' role towards supporting children's emotional recovery, recognizes the value of non-specialist involvement in children's everyday activities. Children's 'crisis' talk or disclosure of traumatic events, when initiated or supported by non-specialists such as teachers, has similarities and differences to how specialist therapists support children (Bateman et al., 2015). There are similarities in that specialists and non-specialists can prompt storytelling about an event, but there are also differences in that teachers and children can display connections through collaborative sharing of events that both have experienced. Further, teachers were more often present and could wait until the moment children spontaneously initiated topics of concern.

Through providing opportunities for children to contribute their voice in everyday interactions, their social competence in managing the recovery process through producing 'tellable' accounts (Bateman et al., 2013a, b) and their role in the co-production of making sense of the disaster through storytelling (Bateman & Danby, 2013) becomes evident.

Professional Reflection

By Paula Robinson and Claire Lethaby
New Brighton Preschool, Christchurch, NZ

Our Story

We want to share with you our story, that is, the story of New Brighton Community Preschool and Nursery, an early childhood centre situated in the eastern suburbs of Christchurch. To share our story we need to set the scene, to tell you a little about who we are and what we experienced but then focus on what we are fairly proud of, that being some of the positive new learning and learning pathways.

The Impact of the Earthquake on the Teachers, Whānau and Children

New Brighton Community Preschool and Nursery was established in 1979 in our eastern, seaside community. We are a not for profit early childhood centre which has always worked proactively for both our children and whānau with whom we proudly work alongside. We experienced four significant earthquakes which also caused closure for varying time periods, added to this were two potential tsunami warnings, a three week period of our road being closed due to potential flooding (luckily for us that stopped two houses away) and the final closure time resulting after two heavy snowfalls! Over this period, our families have had to contend with 41 days of emergency closures, none of which we ever envisaged. At this time, we had 68 families that attended our centre, with children aged from five months through to five years old. Each individual child has undertaken this journey in their own unique style; however, our intention is to portray the main practices which have emerged over this time.

The September 2010 earthquake occurred while we were all home in our beds. While it was a huge experience, it really did not impact on us as directly as subsequent earthquakes. The centre was closed for a couple of days while it was structurally checked, all that occurred was a broom fell over. It did bring a huge awareness to our team and we ensured that practices and procedures in relation to earthquakes were robust. We also ensured that we had appropriate survival kits, even though many of us believed at the time this was a once in a lifetime experience. The children appeared to view the centre as a 'safe place' and maybe this was due to the earthquake occurring outside centre hours. Conversations and practices around the earthquake emerged during children's play, particularly around the shaking feeling, the noise and how it made their bodies feel.

At our teachers' only day at the beginning of 2011, our team went through our environment looking at the safest places for protection in an 'event' and also looking to eliminate any potential hazards. We felt it worthwhile to undertake this exercise together as we had two new teachers and wanted the whole team to hold the same knowledge and information.

It was only two weeks later that the February earthquake occurred. This one was serious, and we evacuated the building to our safest place, which was a lawn area in the back of the preschool playground. Our designated 'assembly point' which we used when practising drills had a power line dangling across it, so immediately we had to alter our plans. Initially there were a lot of children who needed cuddles, but in a short period of time a sing-a-long had begun which gave it a picnic type atmosphere. This went on for over an hour while parents were arriving to collect their treasures. Throughout this time, the ground kept rumbling and shaking and our biggest focus was that the children were ok and that the parents, as they arrived, got the support they needed. Many parents had to abandon their cars on roads that were not driveable and make their way on foot, waddling through liquefaction and flooding, sometimes up to their waist. The one thing we will never forget was the look of relief when they saw their child sitting safely in a teacher's arms. To this day, it still it brings a lump to the throat whenever we think back to it. We stayed on our little grass patch for just over three hours until the last parent arrived.

Initiating Talk About the Earthquakes with the Children

The immediate effects of this quake were the loss of essential services, namely water, power, sewerage and phone. The roads within our community were barely driveable and all shops were closed. This was a change that was forced upon everyone, you had no choice. While some left the area (permanently, or just to escape for a bit), many stayed and tried to get on with adjusting to the new 'normal'. The word which became part of every child's vocabulary was liquefaction. Everyone was in survival mode and really went back to the basics. Children learnt that through crazy hard times, they could continue to live and play, just in a less expectant way. This is something that is a valuable attribute, one which many people in life never learn, but these children have, and they will carry with them this knowledge and know-how for life.

Following the February quake, the Centre Manager attended a Ministry of Education workshop focused on Traumatic Events. A key insight from this workshop was to acknowledge what children were sharing from their perspectives and how it felt, but when ending the conversation trying to incorporate what were the good things that happened at and after this time? ('I was feeling really scared but I got to have a snuggle in bed with mummy'.) This concept guided our belief about acknowledging the difficulty/hardship/challenge/uncertainty/fear, but in our environment, we could also acknowledge the positives, which were and are unique to this situation. We were very aware to hold these conversations with children, this situation was real and affecting their lives, if we talked about with them, maybe it could support them to make sense, meaning or understanding and alleviate some fears.

From this belief, we built a philosophy which was to 'keep it positive' for children. Subsequently, before we came back in March 2011 after the five-week February closure, we had already reflected and discussed at length the ways in which teachers could support our children. Having this foundation knowledge and shared understanding set the scene for making the most of those teachable moments and supporting children in making sense of what was happening in our community.

Importance of Going Out into the Environment

We came back to a new 'normal'. Instead of toilets, we had port-a-loos outside in the entrance foyer, all taps had the heads removed and we used no running water (due to the water still being unsafe to drink). Children had to come with drink bottles of boiled water and hand washing consisted of sanitizer, wipes and more sanitizer. This all seemed like a big ask, but every child and family turned up on our re-opening day. Everyone was desperate to get back to their normal routines and the children appeared keen to get back to their friends and play. Immediately we noticed a change in children's play. We now had experts in road works, drain layers, GNS scientists, builders and port-a-loo cleaners, just to name a few. The immediate environment was offering a rich curriculum of experiences and knowledge. There was a new-found respect and awareness for people in 'day-glow' jackets, particularly the men and women who worked tirelessly outside our houses and always made time to explain what they were doing.

A new learning pathway had emerged over this time and this was an awareness of our ever-changing environment. Around us were continuous roadworks and work on water and sewerage pipes. This was such a rich experience right at our doorsteps and was far too valuable an opportunity to pass up. We made a conscious decision to take the children out to see what was happening in our neighbourhood. Nearly daily we would set off down the road to see the latest happening. We walked with the children and made the effort to point out specific parts of the environment that were damaged and talked to the children about it, asking questions that we hoped would prompt their thinking and understanding. The children were soon creating their own working theories on why something needed replacing or how. The physical environment also created new challenges and that was the flooding that occurred at the end of our street. Our street backs onto the river and with high tides and high water levels, flooding would regularly occur. This again became a site of investigation and the children would note where the flooding was, by taking photos of the mailbox where it was up to, and then come back to the centre to document it all.

Documenting the Earthquake in Learning Stories

These observations and photos were documented in wall displays, which were in the children's play space at their level. Each day the new photo was added to the display as well as children's voices about what they had just observed. This became a great site for children revisiting what they had previously noticed and whether it was similar or different to what they had observed that day. It became a record of what was changing around us and we felt empowered; we weren't sitting back waiting for things to happen to us we were actively noticing what was happening and creating new working theories. Teachers were also busy documenting individual children's ideas and perspectives in their learning stories. At the time, learning stories were either group stories, which shared these experiences and events, or individual stories, which were focused on individual children's perspectives. These stories within their learning journey books were a valuable tool for children to revisit with their peers, teachers and whānau both in the centre and at home.

The main focus within these learning stories was acknowledging and celebrating the competence that the children demonstrated at this challenging time. Having photo displays throughout our learning environment of our community and its ever-changing appearance, as well as many learning stories based on key topics around these experiences, meant the conversations were very rich within the environment and often child initiated. Most children were coming in daily, ready to share their own home experiences with their friends and teachers, bringing new knowledge, comparing stories and experiences, then practising and trialling these in their play. We intentionally provided resources, such as florescent vests, hard hats, road cones and clipboards, to support the theme of their play. Teachers were very mindful to follow children's leads in these conversations. At times conversations served to consolidate learning and ideas. However, teachers were also very mindful to be respectful and sensitive as children had their own experiences of these events.

The June earthquake again occurred while we were at the centre. The first was strong enough to make us evacuate outside and parents again started to come and collect their children. When the second occurred, which was a lot stronger, we only had three children left and a few teachers. The children were soon gone and it was saddening to drive home seeing the broken roads and the liquefaction again. The centre re-opened a week later and we once again welcomed back the children and families. Much of the initial conversations and play was about the earthquakes and the effects these had on each individual's situation. The children talked like experts about their houses and land, what worked and what didn't work and the appearance of any new cracks in buildings. They also began to identify the symbols that had now become part of their community. Examples of these include the Red/Yellow/Green stickers and the many different roadwork signs within the area. The children really identified with these signs knowing what each meant and the actions required; again valuable learning sites within our local environment.

In Conclusion

The word resilience is synonymous with Christchurch and one that we like to try to find other words for. This is our unique story, why use such a common word? However, resilience must be acknowledged. You cannot go through so much repetition of challenge and remain unaffected. We don't believe in the theory that children will just bounce back on their own. We believe that if a child has experienced repeated challenges, yet throughout these challenges their voices are heard, acknowledged and supported, resilience can develop. To gain this disposition, children also need supportive learning partners: peers, parents, neighbours, significant adults and whānau members, not to mention teachers.

We are not wearing 'rose-tinted' glasses when writing this. We acknowledge that this story comes from an early childhood 'centre' perspective. We also recognize that, as teachers, we were not and are not there at all critical times, such as when a child may not want to go to bed at night or may not want to use the toilet because they are scared. This is our 'centre' story and focuses on the positive learning, which we as a teaching team have recognized, acknowledged and focused upon.

References

Arminen, I. (2004). Second stories: The salience of interpersonal communication for mutual help in alcoholics anonymous. *Journal of Pragmatics, 36,* 319–347.

Bateman, A., & Church, A. (2017). Children's use of objects in an early years playground. *European Early Childhood Education Research Journal, 25*(1), 55–71.

Bateman, A., & Danby, S. (2013). Recovering from the earthquake: Early childhood teachers and children collaboratively telling stories about their experiences. *Disaster Management and Prevention Journal, 22*(5), 467–479.

Bateman, A., Danby, S., & Howard, J. (2013a). Everyday preschool talk about Christchurch earthquakes. *Australian Journal of Communication, 40*(1), 103–123.

Bateman, A., Danby, S., & Howard, J. (2013b). Living in a broken world: How young children's well-being is supported through playing out their earthquake experiences. *International Journal of Play, 2*(3), 202–219.

Bateman, A., Danby, S., & Howard, J. (2015). Using conversation analysis for understanding children's talk about traumatic events. In M. O'Reilly & J. Lester (Eds.), *Handbook of child mental health: Discourse and conversation studies* (pp. 402–421). London: Palgrave.

Bateman, A., Danby, S., & Howard, J. (2016). Living in a broken world: How young children's well-being is supported through playing out their earthquake experiences. In C. D. Clark (Ed.), *Play and well being* (pp. 202–219). Oxon: Routledge.

Brown, R. (2012). Principles guiding practice and responses to recent community disasters in New Zealand. *New Zealand Journal of Psychology, 40*(4), 86–89.

Carr, M., & Lee, W. (2012). *Learning stories: Constructing learner identities in early education.* London: Sage.

Cekaite, A. (2010). Shepherding the child: Embodied directive sequences in parent-child interactions. *Text & Talk, 30*(1), 1–25.
Danby, S., Butler, C. W., & Emmison, M. (2011). 'Have you talked with a teacher yet?': How helpline counsellors support young callers being bullied at school. *Children and Society, 25*(4), 328–339.
Dean, S. (2012). Long term support in schools and early childhood services after February 2011. *New Zealand Journal of Psychology, 40*(4), 95–97.
Ekberg, S., Danby, S., Houen, S., Davidson, C., & Thorpe, K. J. (2017). Soliciting and pursuing suggestions: Practices for contemporaneously managing student-centred and curriculum–focused activities. *Linguistics and Education, 42,* 65–73.
Gibbs, L., Mutch, C., O'Connor, P., & MacDougall, C. (2013). Research with, by, for and about children: Lessons from disaster contexts. *Global Studies of Childhood, 3*(2), 129–141.
Goodwin, C. (2017). *Co-operative action.* Cambridge: Cambridge University Press.
Goodwin, M. H. (2006). *The hidden life of girls: Games of stance, status and exclusion.* London: Wiley.
Graffam Walker, A. (2013). *Handbook on questioning children: A linguistic perspective.* Washington, DC: American Bar Association.
Heritage, J. (1984). *Garfinkel and ethnomethodology.* Oxford: Polity Press.
Houen, S., Danby, S., Farrell, A., & Thorpe, K. (2016a). Creating spaces for children's agency: 'I wonder …' formulations in teacher-child interactions. *International Journal of Early Childhood, 48*(3), 259–276.
Houen, S., Danby, S., Farrell, A., & Thorpe, K. (2016b). 'I wonder what you know …': Teachers designing requests for factual information. *Teaching and Teacher Education, 59,* 68–78.
Hutchby, I. (2001). 'Witnessing': The use of first-hand knowledge in legitimating lay opinions on talk radio. *Discourse Studies, 3*(4), 481–497.
Jefferson, G. (2004). Glossary of transcript symbols with an introduction. In G. H. Lerner (Ed.), *Conversation analysis: Studies from the first generation* (pp. 13–23). Philadelphia: John Benjamins.
Ministry of Education. (1996/2017). *Te Whāriki. He Whāriki Mātauranga mō ngā Mokopuna o Aotearoa. Early childhood curriculum.* Wellington, New Zealand: Learning Media.
National Institute of Clinical Excellence (NICE). (2005). *Post-traumatic stress disorder: The management of PTSD in adults and children in primary and secondary care.* National Institute for Clinical Excellence, London: BPS Publications.
New Zealand Police. (2012). http://www.police.govt.nz/list-deceased.

O'Connor, P. (2012). *Applied theatre: Aesthetic pedagogies in a crumbling world.* London: Routledge.

Pink, S. (2013). *Doing visual ethnography.* London: Sage.

Prendiville, E. (2014). Abreaction. In C. Schaefer & A. Drewes (Eds.), *The therapeutic powers of play: 20 core agents of change.* Hoboken, NJ: Wiley.

Ruf, M., Schauer, M., Neuner, F., Catani, C., Schauer, E., & Elbert, T. (2010). Narrative exposure therapy for 7- to 16-year-olds: A randomised controlled trial with traumatized refugee children. *Journal of Traumatic Stress, 24*(3), 437–445.

Sacks, H. (1984). On doing "being ordinary". In J. M. Atkinson & J. Heritage (Eds.), *Structures of social action: studies in conversation analysis* (pp. 413–440). Cambridge: Cambridge University Press and Editions de la Maison des Sciences de l'Homme.

Sacks, H. (1992). *Lectures on conversation* (G. Jefferson, Trans. Vols. I & II). Oxford, UK: Blackwell.

Sacks, H., Schegloff, E. A., & Jefferson, G. (1974). A simplest systematics for the organization of turn-taking in conversation. *Language, 50*(4), 696–735.

Schegloff, E. A. (1968). Sequencing in conversational openings. *American Anthropologist* [New Series], *70*(6), 1075–1095.

Schegloff, E. A. (1980). Preliminaries to preliminaries "Can I ask you a question." *Sociological Enquiry, 50* (3–4), 104–152.

Schegloff, E. A. (2007). Sequence organisation in interaction: A primer in conversational analysis (Vol. 1). Cambridge: Cambridge University Press.

5

Misleading the Alleged Offender: Child Witnesses' Displays of Competence in Police Interviews

Guusje Jol, Wyke Stommel and Wilbert Spooren

Professional Reflection by Naomi Dessaur

Introduction

In this chapter, we analyze police interrogations with children who have been witness of a sexual offense. Such interviews are likely to be difficult for the child. The reason for the interrogation is a crisis that often involves an alleged offender who is known to them. The physical setting of the interview is unfamiliar to the children and they have to talk to a relative stranger about potentially traumatic and sometimes taboo events.

G. Jol (✉) · W. Stommel · W. Spooren
Centre for Language Studies, Radboud University Nijmegen, Nijmegen, The Netherlands
e-mail: g.jol@let.ru.nl

W. Stommel
e-mail: w.stommel@let.ru.nl

J. Lamerichs et al. (eds.), *Children and Mental Health Talk*, The Language of Mental Health,
https://doi.org/10.1007/978-3-030-28426-8_5

The relationship with their conversational partner is asymmetrical in the sense that the interlocutor determines the agenda and what counts as a good answer. In sum, the children find themselves in an extremely difficult situation. We will demonstrate that children nevertheless turn out to be competent communicators who are capable both of managing the local interaction and of reporting coherently about a difficult situation.

Children as Reliable Witnesses

The question whether children are capable interlocutors is very salient in the context of criminal investigations. For a long time, children were regarded as too unreliable to testify as witnesses (Goodman, 1984). However, research has shown that children can be reliable witnesses, especially if they are interviewed in a way that encourages children to tell their own story and police officers avoid leading and suggestive questioning as much as possible (e.g., Lamb, Orbach, Hershkowitz, Esplin, & Horowitz, 2007). This way of interviewing has been put forward in various guidelines, trainings and protocols for investigative interviewing. This holds specifically for instructions for the cases that we will discuss in this chapter, namely interviewing child victims of alleged sexual assault. These guidelines also emphasize the importance of building rapport and being supportive. For example, in case children are quiet or emotional, police officers are encouraged to ask what is happening so that they can help the child (revised NICHD protocol 2014, http://nichdprotocol.com/), presumably to address feelings of distress. Relevant guidelines are, for example, the Achieving Best Evidence (ABE) guideline by the Ministry of Justice in England and Wales 2011, the National Institute of Child and Health Development (NICHD) protocol in the USA (Lamb et al., 2007 and its revised version 2014) and the Dutch manual for interviewing children (Dekens & van der Sleen, 2013: 47–48; see for concise overviews: Fogarty, Augoustinos, & Kettler, 2013; Jakobsen, Langballe, & Schultz, 2017). Interviews that follow such guidelines can, therefore, be regarded as

---

W. Spooren
e-mail: w.spooren@let.ru.nl

an opportunity for children to tell their story to someone who takes them seriously. In a report by Defence for Children, some children report feeling relieved after the interview (Hokwerda, Veldman, de Graaf, & Rueb, 2015: 66, 71). Research has also shown that investigative interviews can even have therapeutic effects: the child might feel acknowledged when heard (for a brief overview: Jakobsen et al., 2017: 428).

Nevertheless, the interview presents child witnesses with a potentially difficult situation for three main reasons. First, children are expected to talk about a topic that they likely find difficult to discuss, such as sexual violence or other severe cases of violence. It is likely to be even more difficult to talk about these topics with a stranger, despite all efforts to build rapport and be supportive. It may be especially difficult if the alleged offender is someone familiar to the child, as is often the case in sexual violence cases (National Rapporteur, 2014: 78–79). Second, police interviews are not supportive by nature. The institutional goal of investigative interviews is truth finding or fact finding. It is, therefore, the task for the police officer to critically investigate whether something happened that warrants criminal investigation. Hence, police officers need to ask critical follow-up questions and be careful not to go along with the victim's[1] story too quickly (e.g., Antaki, Richardson, Stokoe, & Willott, 2015b: 331; Dekens & van der Sleen, 2013: 71, 100–101; Luchjenbroers & Aldridge, 2013: 309). Some children indeed evaluate this factual approach as problematic afterward, even when they claim to understand why such questioning is necessary (Hokwerda et al., 2015: 81–82).

Third, special measures that aim at ensuring the reliability of interviews with child witnesses can also lead to a less 'friendly' interview for the child, however well-intended the measures may be. For example, police officers are trained to interview children as neutrally and objectively as possible, that is, without being suggestive and influencing the witness' testimony (Dekens & van der Sleen, 2013). Yet, Jakobsen et al. (2017) have shown that such attempts to be neutral sometimes go at the expense of the supportiveness of the interview. The study showed Norwegian police

[1]We are aware of voices that advocate the term 'survivor' rather than 'victim', because the former is a more empowering term (Kelly, 1988). However, we will follow the terms 'victim' and 'witness' because that is the usual terminology in the Netherlands.

officers recordings of their own interviews with child witnesses in distress. The police officers regularly commented that they had been so focused on their task to be neutral that this led to being less than optimally supportive. Such lack of support may even come across to some as child-*un*friendly (Van der Kruis, 2014). Interactional studies of investigative interviews with children have pointed out that there is a tension between collecting evidence in a neutral way on the one hand and being supportive on the other (Childs & Walsh, 2017; Iversen, 2018).

In this chapter, we aim to show how child victims and child witnesses of sexual violence establish being both competent victims and witnesses during the offense and how that contributes to narratives that are robust in the face of damaging kinds of reasoning. Hence these reports can be viewed as one way in which children display being competent interactants, despite the difficulties mentioned above. More specifically, we look at children's reports of misleading the alleged offender.

Saying 'No'

One piece of advice to potential target groups of sexual violence is to 'say no' and to say 'I don't want that'. Kitzinger and Frith (1999) point out that rape prevention programs often include advice to refuse in such direct and explicit ways. The authors argue that this is problematic because the responsibility of avoiding unwanted sex is placed on the victim, rather than on the alleged offender. This is even more problematic because conversation analytic research has shown that the social norm for refusals in everyday life is to produce them as dispreferred turns, that is, *in*directly and *with* accounts. Often, refusals do not even include the word 'no'. For instance, saying 'I'm very busy now' can accomplish a refusal. Moreover, speakers usually avoid damaging relationships by claiming that they are unable rather than unwilling to comply. The authors suggest that the advice 'just to say no' is not a good advice, as it conflicts with cultural norms (Kitzinger & Frith, 1999: 203).

Kitzinger and Frith (1999; Frith & Kitzinger, 1997) also asked female school and university students in focus groups to talk about how to refuse sex. The participants reported to find it inappropriate and difficult to just say no. Therefore, the authors argue that this can be taken as a sign of having acquired the cultural and interactional norm that refusals are usually performed indirectly and implicitly, even though 'feminist and date rape prevention literatures [...] present such refusals as inadequate and insufficiently communicative' (Kitzinger & Frith, 1999). They conclude that the claim that alleged offenders may misunderstand an indirect refusal of sex is highly implausible, as this is the normal way refusals are done.

Kitzinger and Frith's (1999) argument is relevant for the topic of children's reports of having misled or attempted to mislead the alleged offender. It suggests that being indirect in a situation of abuse, for example by misleading the alleged offender, is a display of interactional competence. Additionally, the report inevitably functions within the interactional context of the police interview and thus performs actions toward the police officer (cf. Schegloff, 1997; see also Fogarty, 2010: 310–313). In this chapter, we investigate the interrelated questions of how reports of misleading portray the child in the reported offence and what that establishes in the police interview.

Context: Dutch Police Interviews with Child Witnesses

Dutch police interviews with children take place in special child-friendly interview rooms. These interview rooms have been furnished to make the child feel at ease and they are equipped with cameras and microphones to record both the child and the police officer during the interview (Ministerie van Veiligheid en Justitie, 2013). The main purpose of these recordings is to make the original interview available for the police, prosecutors, lawyers, expert witnesses and, ultimately, judges (Ministerie van Veiligheid en Justitie, 2013). However, police officers point out that prosecutors, defense lawyers and the court usually do not watch the recordings. Instead, transcripts and summaries are made and added to the case file. These documents then serve as the basis for the judge's verdict. Only when requested or if there is doubt about the interview techniques, parts of the interview may be played in court. Police officers generally try to interview a child only once, in order to minimalize the burden on the child

(Dekens & van der Sleen, 2013: 56; Hokwerda et al., 2015) and to reduce the possibility that the interviews change the child's recollection of what happened (Dekens & van der Sleen, 2013: 47, 71, 105).

The interviews in the dataset are one-on-one encounters between a police officer and a child.[2] Children aged up to eleven years old must be interviewed in a child-friendly interview room (Ministerie van Veiligheid en Justitie, 2013).[3] Police officers refer to these interviews as interviews with child witnesses, even though many of them are direct victims of the alleged abuse.

Police officers are trained to interview children according to the 'scenario model'. This model has been developed by the Dutch police academy and is based on the trainers' experience and research (Dekens & van der Sleen, 2013). It aims at avoiding suggestive questioning and suggestion in general. Like other guidelines for investigative interviewing (ABE, NICHD protocol), the model involves several phases: an introduction phase, a phase of giving instructions or ground rules (e.g., that the child should correct the police officer when necessary), a free narrative or free recall phase (when the child does the talking and the police officer listens), a questioning phase (when the police officer elicits more details about the story) and a closure phase (when the police officer thanks the child and gives the child the opportunity to ask questions [but see for a discussion of this opportunity Childs & Walsh, 2018]).

Data and Method

This study is part of a research project to examine how advice literature on police interviews with children and the actual interviews relate to each other (see also Jol & Stommel, 2016a, 2016b). The materials used for this chapter are 30 audiovisual recordings made by the police in two child-friendly interview rooms in 2011 and 2012. The interviews used for the

[2]Exceptions to this rule are interviews with an interpreter, and very rare occasions when a caregiver can be present.

[3]Hokwerda et al. (2015) have argued in their Defence for Children Report that all minors (people under 18) who are victims of an alleged crime should be interviewed in the child-friendly interview room by a certified police officer.

analysis were selected on the basis of criteria such as age and gender, the nature of the alleged offense, the year of recording and the absence of an interpreter. We also asked not to include high profile or 'spectacular' cases to avoid interference with such publicized cases and to demonstrate that we were not sensation seeking. For the recordings from one child-friendly interview room, the first author sat together with a police officer to select recordings. For the recordings from the second child-friendly interview room, the first author sent a list of criteria to the police. The police sent a list of interviews that was slightly revised after questions of the first author.

The data are naturally occurring materials in the sense that the recordings were already made for the criminal investigation without intervention by the researchers. The children (eleven boys and nineteen girls) are between six and eleven years old. The materials have been obtained with permission of the public prosecutor's office and with cooperation of the police. Only the transcripts have been anonymized; the videos were only accessible to the authors of this chapter and were stored in a safe. Using materials that were not collected for research purposes raises all sorts of ethical issues. These issues have been discussed in detail with the police, the public prosecutor and with the faculty's Ethics Assessment Committee. This has resulted in approval from the parties involved. A detailed discussion of these considerations can be found in Jol and Stommel (2016b).

It struck us that children regularly produce accounts of their own role in the event that were unsolicited by the police officer. Some of these accounts include reports of resistance by misleading the alleged offender. In this chapter, we focus on accounts of misleading the alleged offender, both volunteered and invited. We are interested in what children establish with such an account, both in the reported event and, consequently, in the interview. We screened verbatim transcripts for children describing their own conduct in relation to the alleged offender in terms that imply that they misled the alleged offender. This included 'trick' (*truc/trucje*), 'to pretend' (*doen alsof*), 'pulling someone's leg' (*in de maling nemen*) and 'making excuses' (*smoesjes*). We also included a few less explicit fragments about children saying or doing something potentially untrue when or because they want to get away from the alleged offender. We identified thirteen instances from eight different interviews, conducted by six different police officers. The fragments identified were transcribed using Jeffersonian transcription conventions for conversation analysis (CA) (Jefferson,

2004) and, when relevant, using transcription conventions for embodied behavior and CA as developed by Mondada (2014). Fragments are presented in Dutch with an English translation that is a compromise between literal translation and maintaining the flow of the talk.

The children in the collection are all girls, in the age of seven (two children), eight (two children), nine (one child), ten (two children) and eleven (one child). All interviews concern an alleged sex crime, but the sexual violence in these instances varies in nature. The collection includes both children who were witness to a single offense (six interviews) or to a series of offenses (two interviews). Producing claims of misleading the offender is not a very common practice because the goals of these police interview do not make such claims relevant, i.e., the police's questions are usually not directed at finding out whether the child misled the alleged offender. Hence, the fact that in eight of the thirty interviews, children make such claims indicates a clear importance of raising this issue from the perspective of quite a few children.

Analysis: Reports of Misleading

In this section, we discuss four examples of children who report how they misled the suspect or attempted to mislead the suspect. In the first two fragments, the report involves a single event; in the third and fourth fragment, the children report strategies adopted in a series of events.

The first fragment is taken from an interview with Jentl (7).[4] In the fragment, the interviewee reports that she and her friend Wencke (8) were playing outside when an unknown man pulled Wencke on his lap and rubbed her belly. Prior to the fragment, Jentl has reported that the man did so twice: first near the flat where one of the girls lives, and somewhat later on the same day in a nearby park. The fragment is taken from the questioning phase and concerns how the second instance ended. The police officers' speech is indicated with a P and the children's speech is indicated with a K throughout the analysis. Note that the translations are as literal as possible.

[4]Throughout the analyses we follow the convention that ages of the children are indicated by numbers in parentheses.

Fragment 1: Jentl (7) 26 minutes: so she could get off his lap

```
1   P:     =.hh en hoe <st↑opt> dat #dan#,
           =.hh and how {does} that stop then,
2          die tweede #keer#,
           that second #time#,
3   K: →   e:h;
           e:h;
4          (0.9)
5      →   uhm toen zei ik .h zullen we varen,=
           uhm then I said .h shall we go sailing,=
6          =en toen zei die .h meneer nog één minuut;
           =and then that .h mister said one more minute;
7          (0.4)
8          nog een paar telletjes;
           another few seconds;
9      →   en toen .h zei ik;
           and then .h I said;
10     →   ↑dan zullen we dan nu gaan?=
           ↑shall we go now then?=
11         =en toen .H toen (0.3) zei die men'-
           =and then .H then (0.3) that mist'-
11         toen toe we bij e:h (.) bij de flat weer waren,=
           when we were near e:h (.) the flat again,=
13         =zei die niet tegen je ouders vertellen.
           =he said don't tell your parents.
14  P:     okee;=
           okay;=
15         =.H dus jIJ komt-jij zegt dan op een g'even moment tegen
           =.H so yOU come-you say then at a certain moment to
16         Wencke;=
           Wencke;=
17         =zullen we gaan <varen>?
           =shall we go <sailing>?
18         .h w↑↑AArom zei je dat ↓tegen °°Wencke°°;
           .h w↑↑HY did you say that to °°Wencke°°;
19         (0.5)
20  K: →   omdat ik-
           because I-
21         (1.2)
22     →   omdat (.) zij dan van die meneer z'n schoot af k.hh kon,=
           because (.) she could go off that mister's lap then,=
23     →   =want ik dacht al aan haar gezicht,
           =because I already thought on her face,
24     →   dat ze- .h dat ze `t niet wou;
           that she- .h that she didn't want it;
```

```
25       → en dat ze 't niet durfde.
           and that she didn't dare it.
26   P:    ok↑ee,=
           o:k↑ee,=
27         =.h je dacht,
           =.h you thought,
28         aan haar gezicht,
           on her face,
29         aan ↑Wencke gezi- d'r gezicht te zien,=
           on ↑Wencke seen- her face to see,=
           you thought that you could see on her face
30         =.hh ↓ dat ze 't niet leuk vond;
           =.hh ↓ that she didn't like it;
31         en dat ze 't °niet°- dat ze nie wilde,
           and that she didn't - that she did not want {it},
32         .H en daarom bedach jij van;
           .H and that's why you thought of like
33         (0.5)
34         te zeggen;
           saying;
35         (0.3)
36         zullen we gaan varen .
           shall we go sailing.
```

Jentl first responds to the police officer's question (lines 1–2) that she proposed to go sailing (she tells elsewhere that her friend Wencke has a small boat) (lines 3–5). She reports that this proposal was not immediately successful: the man did not let her friend go immediately (lines 6–8). She reports pursuing her attempt (lines 9–10) and the juxtaposed phrase 'when we were near the flat again' (line 12) implies that her second proposal was successful. The police officer acknowledges this answer with 'okay' (line 14) and displays reception with a partitial answer repetition (lines 15–17). This answer-repetition is then coupled with a *why*-question: 'why did you say that to Wencke?' (line 18). This question establishes that the police officer does not accept the child's story straightaway, solicits a reason and therefore claims that Jentl's reported proposal to go sailing does not make immediate sense. The officer's questions could thus be heard as taking a critical stance (Bolden & Robinson, 2011; see also Sacks, 1995: 4–5, 72–80).

Jentl begins her answer with a delay and 'because I' (line 20), yet she abandons this answer and changes the sentence subject into 'she' after another delay. This downplays her own wishes and present her move as altruistic: she said it to provide *her friend* with an opportunity to get off the alleged offender's lap (line 23). Moreover, her response reconstructs her previous reported proposal to go sailing as something she said *in order to* help her friend. The account solicitation thus elicits a reconstruction of Jentl's previous report of a proposal to go sailing into an *excuse* to get away from the man. The police officer receives this response as causing a shift in understanding by rising intonation in 'okay' (line 26) the emphatic 'and that's why' (line 32), thus retrospectively constructing the *why*-account as seeking an explanation rather than challenging Jentl's telling as well as treating the child's reported motivation and strategy as important and relevant.

Jentl also warrants her attempt to help by referring to her friend's facial expression (lines 23–25). This portrays her as knowing her friend well enough to understand from a facial expression what she is thinking. The warrant further constructs the proposal she came up with in the face of the alleged abuse, i.e., at the moment she could read in her friends face that she 'didn't want it and didn't dare it' (lines 24–25). The proposal is put forward as an ad hoc strategy to deal with this particular incident.

In retrospect, then, the police officer's *why*-question enables Jentl to present herself in a favorable way. She assumes a role of a having correctly identified her friend's problem, having acted upon that understanding of the situation and having resisted the alleged offender *in the reported event* by offering her friend a way out of the situation using her wit and knowledge of her friend. She thus establishes having been a capable and helpful friend during the event. Importantly, this portrayal is situated in the ongoing police interview. As such, it contributes to a narrative of what happened that counters other versions of the story (cf. Potter, 1996: 106–108), and particular versions in which she did *not* resist. Such a version would be vulnerable to potential undermining and blame-attributing questions like 'but why didn't you help your friend?' (cf. questions to the alleged victim Antaki et al., 2015a). Hence, the current version of the story "pre-empts and mitigates potential blame implications" (MacLeod, 2016: 108) that might occur later in the criminal proceedings or in the police interview.

The girl in the next fragment, 10-year-old Merel, also constructs a proposal in order to physically exit the situation and close down the interaction with the alleged offender. Different from Fragment 1, this fragment is taken from the free recall phase of the interview. The construction is produced in an extended turn rather than in response to a question from the interviewer (as in Fragment 1). Therefore, it can be considered unsolicited.

The police officer invites Merel to talk (lines 1–3), and she explains (lines omitted) that she was at her friend's place and her friend, Thije, was doing something on the computer. The boy's father was there too and invited her to sit. Merel reports that she refused and that her friend's father then puts her jokingly on his lap. The fragment continues when the father starts touching her (line 30). The police officer is writing throughout most of the fragment. The excuse starts in line 42. Non-capital p's and k's in the transcript indicate embodied behavior during the other participant's speech.

Fragment 2: Merel (10) 9 minutes: because I wanted that that father would stop that;

```
1    P:    %.hhhh nOU (.) Merelh;
            .hhhh wELL (.) Merel;
           %writes--->
2          (1.0)%
           ---->%
3          wat kom °jij mij° vertellen,
           what have you come to tell me,
```

((26 lines omitted))

```
30   K:    en (.) toen eerst ging die onder m'n shirt voelen enzo;
           and (.) then first he went feeling under my shirt and stuff
           like that;
```

((8 lines ommitted in which K tells how her friend's father goes up with his hand and then in her pants, panties and in her crotch))

```
39   K:    >en toen ging die ook zegmaar<;=
           >and then he also did like<;=
40         =overal voelen enzo;
           =feel everywhere and stuff like that;
41         (0.8)
42       → •pt en: (.) eh daarna vroeg ik aan Thije:
           •pt and (.) eh after that I asked Thije:
43         (0.2)
44       → eh zegmaar van;
           eh say like;
```

```
45        → ↓°das mijn  %vriendje°                       ;=
            ↓°that's my %little friend/boyfriend5° ;=
    p:                  %nods while writing-->
47  K:      =.hhh% °ehm° van-(0.2) e:hm;-
            =.hhh% °ehm° like-(0.2) ehm;-
    p:      ---->%
48          (0.9)
49  K:  →   zullen wij naar bUIten gaan?=
            shall we go OUTside?=
50      →   =want ik wou      dat  die   vader [daarmee] ophoudde;
            =because I wanted that that father that he would stop that;
51  P:                                         [hmhm    ]
                                               [hmhm    ]
52  K:  →   ↓°maar dat durfde ik niet-niet te zeggen,
            ↓°but I didn't-not dare to say that
53          .hh
            .hh
54          (0.3)
55          •pt enne toen zei die  ja: okee ,=
            •pt and eh then he said  jeah okay ,=
```

[5] *Vriendje* is a diminutive of *vriend* ('friend'). In Dutch it is often used as 'boyfriend', but given that they are both children, it can also be used as 'little friend'.

Like Jentl in Fragment 1, Merel reports a proposal to get away from the alleged offender (lines 42–45, 49–50, 52). She accounts for this strategy by referring to a dilemma of wanting the father to stop (line 50) versus being too scared to say so explicitly (line 52). This claim of having been too scared implies that she in fact did not explicitly tell her friend's father to stop and it warrants for not doing so by claiming that she was to scared. She thus orientates to the lack of an explicit request to stop as something that needs explanation. Hence, she treats explicit requests to stop as something that may be expected. At the same time, Merel presents just saying 'no' or 'stop' as having potential (interactional) repercussions (cf. Kitzinger & Frith, 1999).

The reported dilemma between wanting to stop her friend's father and being scared presents her proposal to go outside as produced in order to escape from the situation and, hence, as an excuse *in order to* escape from the situation and, hence, as an excuse. This leads to a narrative again in which the child resisted the alleged offender even though she did not do so explicitly. This counters versions of the story that are vulnerable to the accusation that she is at fault because she did not provide resistance. Different from Fragment 1, she reports the proposal without a solicitation by the police officer. Her orientation to the norm of resistance is more independently produced than in Fragment 1. This is poignant because apparently the child herself feels the need to make relevant this norm in the context of this police interview, even in the absence of legal or other cues that resistance and blame are an issue. Notice how the fear that is included in the child's account for not directly requesting to let her go (line 52) is sensitive to the same normative orientation. Also note that the police officer could have approved of, or at least acknowledged, Jentl's strategy in lines 53 and 54, but that she remains silent.

Fragment 3 is taken from the questioning phase with Delphine (9). She uses the verb 'pretend to' (*net doen alsof*). This makes her claim explicit that she attempted to mislead the alleged offender. Delphine has asserted in the free recall phase that she has been abused by her father repeatedly and that it lasted for a year and a half. Fragment 3 is taken from an episode in which the police officer invites a narrative of what happened the last time Delphine was abused. The police officer invites the child to continue in line 4, but disrupts her narrative several times to solicit accounts of how Delphine knows (data not shown). The fragment continues with a question by the police officer (line 38) and response by Delphine (lines 39–44). The stretched 'me' (line 44) and the rising intonation, project more talk to come, yet the police officer disrupts her narrative with another request for an account: 'how {do} you know that daddy knows that' (line 45).

Fragment 3: Delphine (9) 51 minutes: so I pretend that I'm in a very deep sleep

```
((P and K are both looking at a map of child's father's house; K
holds map + pen))
1    P:   maar- okee;
          but- okay;
2         papa komt naar je j-die kamer toe: ,
          daddy comes to your y-that room ,
3    K:   ↑hm↑hm?
          ↑hm↑hm?
4    P:   en hoe gaat ut dan verder;
          and how does it continue;
          and what happens next;
5    K:   .hh dan (0.7) °b:°en ik *d↑i:t,                    *
          .hh then (0.7) th↑is is me,
                                  *points with pen on map*

((32 lines omitted))

38   P:   >en% *wanneer WORD JIJ DAN OPGEH↑AALD,
          >and%*when ARE YOU THEN PICKED UP,
          -->%
     k:        *pen on paper------->
39   K:   nou als Berend- als papah playstation hoort,
          well when Berend- when daddy hears playstation,
40        en ye↑:s,
          and ye↑:s,
41        dan weet ie dat >Berend heeft< gescoord;
          he knows that >Berend has scored;
42        met zijn <voet↑bal>,
          with his <football>,
43        .HHH dus.
          .HHH so.
44        dan loopt papa naar <m[ij: >,
          then daddy walks to <me:>,
45   P:                         [hoe weet jij dat papa *dat weet?
                                [how {do} you know that daddy knows
          that?
     k:                                                *looks up-->
46        (0.5)
47   K:   (hh)
48        .hh £omdat ik Berend ook£ ↑Y:ES ↓hoor (0.3) [roepen,
          .hh £because I also£ hear Berend (0.3) shout ↑Y:ES,
49   P:                                               [aukee;
                                                      [okay;
50   K:   en dan:* *weet ik,
          and then  I know,
          ------>* *pen+gaze on paper, writes/draws--->>
```

```
51      dat papa dat dan (kon);=
        that daddy (could) {hear} that then;=
52    → =.hh >dus dan doe ik net alsof da'k in diepe slaap ben;=
        =.hh >so then I pretend that I'm in a deep sleep;=
53      =maar dan maakt ie me wakker<;
        =but then he wakes me up<;
54      .HHH
        .HHH
55      dus dan doe ik,--
        so then I do,--
56      (.)
57      is ↑dit papa.
        is ↑this daddy.
58      (0.6)
59      <nou loo:pt pap°a (0.7) o°ok hierh↑ee:n>?
        <now daddy also walks (0.7) to ↑he:re>
```

Delphine first deals with the *how do you know*-question in lines 47–48, 50–52, presenting the answer as self-evident, which is reinforced by laughter intonation (line 47) and smiley voice (line 48) (cf. Jol & Stommel, 2016a). She claims having heard her brother and unpacks her inference: if she could hear her brother, so could her father (lines 50–51).

She then resumes her narrative with an inbreath and 'so' (*dus*) (line 52) and she claims having consciously attempted to mislead the suspect using 'pretending' (line 54). Additionally, Delphine reports having pretended to be asleep in an intensified way, namely a *deep* sleep (Pomerantz, 1986). This suggests that she did not easily show that she was awake and that she made every effort to keep pretending, in spite of possible attempts to 'wake her up' by her father. She thus strengthens her claim of resistance and thus counters potential a less favorable hearing by the police officer (cf. Pomerantz, 1986).

Different from the previous fragments, Delphine's reported strategy concerns anticipated abuse that she is trying to avoid. She presents her strategy as a way of acting upon knowledge about what will happen when her father wakes up using 'so' (line 52): he will come to her room, so she pretended to be asleep. She has also reported earlier in the interview (data not shown) that she pretended to be asleep after an occasion of abuse. She claims that her father actually fell asleep, which in turn enabled Delphine to remove herself from the situation. The reported strategy in Fragment 3 is thus closely connected to the predictability of her father's behavior and to repeated abuse. The child presents herself as having been a competent victim who anticipated the alleged offender's behavior, even though the strategy was not successful in the end. This, then, pre-empts potential blame-attributing ractions to the story.

The final fragment offers an even more explicit formulation of misleading the alleged offender: the child reports performing a trick. The fragment is taken from the questioning phase of an interview with Dorien (11) about sexual abuse by a family friend named Karel during joint holidays and other social gatherings. After the initial question-answer-uptake sequence (lines 1–4) the police officer asks for clarification whether it happened on the couch or whether she is talking about another occasion now (data not shown). Dorien claims it was another time and then elaborates on those other times: Karel told her to come to his room in the morning. Just prior to line 26 she reports that Karel's wife was in bed too, still sleeping. She then voluntarily reports the trick in line 29.

Fragment 4: Dorien (11) 38 minutes: I have a trick

```
1    P:    .hh (.) heb jij iets (.) bij (1.1) <Karel>(1,5) moeten doen;
           .hh (.) did you (1.5) have to do something (.) to (1.1) <Karel>;
2    K:    *e:h        **£ja: ik moest aan z'n* *piemel zitten£*;
            e:h         £yes I had to touch his willy        £*;
           *gaze away**vague smile           * *  gaze at P     *
3          (0.5)
4    P:    •hh aan z'n piemel zitten;=
           •hh touch his willy;=

 ((19 lines omitted))

26   P:    =↓hm↑hm,
           =↓hm↑hm,
27         (0.2)
28   K:    •hh e:n alleen--
           •hh a:nd only--
29       → *ik heb juist een trucje?=
            I have {juist} a little trick?=
           *smile--------------->
30       → =de: •hh vorige keren,*
           =the •hh previous times,*
           --------------------->*
31       → hebbik juist •h    £net gedaan£
           I  have {juist} •h £pretended £
32       → alsof ik heel lang (0,2) *d↑oor sl↑ie:p?*
           that I kept sleeping very long
                                     *gaze on P      *
```

```
33          [•hhh
            [•hhh
34    P:    [hm↑hm;
            [hm↑hm;
35    K: →  *terw£ij:l 'kgewoon £helemaal wakker was, £*
            *whi£:le I was just totally awake,          £*
            *smile------------------------------------->*
36    P:    [hm↑hm>
            [hm↑hm>
37    K: →  [*maar-i* (.) ik wou niet naar um toe komen?=
            [*but-I * (.) I didn't want to come to him?=
             *smile *
38       →  =•hh 's dee ik net alsof ik £slie:p£;
            =•hh so I pretended to be   £aslee:p£;
39          •hh en dan zei die elke ochtend;
            •hh and then he said every morning;
40          ja: waarom kwam je nie: ;
            yeah why didn't you come;
41          en toe'zei ik;
            and then I said;
42          ja;
            yeah;
43          •hh sorry;
            •hh sorry;
44       →  ik was aan't slapen enzo;
            I was sleeping and stuff like that;
45       →  [terwijl'k gewoon in een boek zat te lezen,
            [while I was just reading in a book,
46    P:    [(hm;)
            [(hm;)
47            [hm↑hm,
              [hm↑hm,
48    K:      [•hh
              [•hh
49          (0.9)
50       →  e::n dan hoefde ik niet (0,4) (<°daar°>)
            a::nd then I didn't have to (0.4) (<that>)
51          (1)
52       →  >aan te zitten zeg maar<;
            >like touch {that}<;
53    P:    °hmhm°;
            °hmhm°;
54          ok#ee#.
            ok#ay#.
55          .hhh daar gaan we `t ↑daalijk samen over hebben,
            .hhh we are going to talk about that together ↑later,
```

Dorien launches her report of misleading the alleged offender with an explicit characterization of what she did: it was a trick. This launch has similar functions to story prefaces (Mandelbaum, 2013; Sacks, 1974): it projects that the 'trick' will be elaborated, and hence that more talk is underway, while also indicating what will be required to bring the story to completion (some instance of being smart must be reported) and to the manner in which a recipient might respond (offering compliments or approval). In lines 30–32, she indeed produces an elaboration of the trick. Like Delphine in Fragment 3, she pretended to be asleep. The addition 'the previous times' suggests that the abuse happened more often and that she has used the trick multiple times. This suggests that the trick has proven to be useful over time. The strategy is also presented as something she is proud of with the word 'trick' and an accompanying smile. The gaze in P's direction when the elaboration is possibly complete (line 32) therefore makes relevant an approving uptake by the police officer.

The police officer, however, does not overtly affiliate with the reported instance of resistance. She could have acknowledged the reported trick in line 33, in overlap with Dorien's inbreath. Instead, she produces a minimal uptake. This lack of uptake can be understood as a way to 'doing being neutral' and thus abide by the guideline to be neutral for this type of interviewing (cf. Antaki et al., 2015c). However, Dorien treats the lack of uptake as problematic and emphasizes that it was a strategy that she adopted in order to avoid the alleged offender (lines 35, 37–45) and that there was a discrepancy between what she said (I was sleeping) and what she was doing (just reading a book).

The strategy is reported as successful: not only was it a way to avoid the alleged offender at the time of the intended abuse, she claims that it also provided her with an excuse when he held her accountable for not following his instructions later on (lines 39–40). She presents this success as something she is proud of with a smile (line 37) and a smiley voice (line 38). At the same time, she leaves the assessment to the police officer, thus adhering to the preference to avoid self-praise (Pomerantz, 1978). The police officer, however, again does not provide such an assessment, despite opportunities in overlap with the inbreath or in pauses (lines 38, 39, 47 and 49). Dorien then further elaborates why exactly she adopted this strategy: so she did not have to touch Karel's private parts. The police officer could have produced a positive evaluation in line 51, anticipating what Dorien projects in line 50. However the police officer remains silent. Dorien then makes explicit what she could avoid by pretending to be asleep, namely touching 'that' (line 52) and in line 53. Again, the police officer only produces a minimal uptake (lines 53–54) and then closes this topic, at least for the time being (line 55).

In the fragment, Dorien uses various means to make relevant an approving uptake: the explicit labels of 'trick' and 'pretending', emphasis, smiles and a smiley voice, and accounts for why she adopted the pretending strategy. She thus presents this strategy as something to be acknowledged and, hence, as the right thing to do. This becomes even more salient by her pursuit of approval. Dorien thus orientates to her own reported behavior as having competently followed a norm of providing resistance. Consequently, Dorien develops a narrative of having well thought out her strategy for managing the abusive situation. This not only counters other, potentially damaging versions of the story, but also constructs her reported behavior as something to be proud of.

Conclusion and Discussion

The analysis shows that, despite several differences, the reports of misleading have in common that they portray the child as having competently and actively resisted the alleged offender at the time of the (attempted) offense. They also manage critical questions (Fragment 1) and are not necessarily taken up in an affiliative way (Fragments 2 and 4). The reports of misleading also present resistance to an alleged offender as something that can be accomplished without overt resistance, by implicit verbal strategies (Fragments 1–2) as well as by embodied behavior (Fragments 3–4). The analysis adds to the argument of Kitzinger and Frith (1999; see also Woodhams, Hollin, Bull, & Cooke, 2012) that even children as young as 7–11 sometimes report the use of other and more face-saving strategies than 'just saying no'. Fragment 2 in particular shows awareness of potential repercussions of explicit and overt resistance (cf. Kitzinger & Frith, 1999).

Inherently, the reports of misleading the offender accomplish interactional work in the interactional setting of the police interview. In Fragment 1, the girl provides a response to the challenging question why she proposed to go sailing, and in Fragment 4, the girl competently pursues an approving uptake. Additionally, the accounts in Fragments 2–4 are significant in that they are unsolicited, hence volunteered by the child. They thus contribute to the narrative of what happened in a certain way, namely by highlighting their resistance (cf. Fogarty, 2010: 278–313). Like any way of constructing a story or account is tailored to counter other versions of the story (Potter, 1996), the children's versions counter competing versions of what happened that possible undermining lines of reasoning in which the child is at fault because the child did not resist (cf. MacLeod, 2016).

It is poignant that some children in our corpus orient to the norm of resistance, even though they are not to be blamed socially or legally. A possible reason why children may make relevant resistance in their talk, why it is recognizable as a favorable portrayal, and why police officer do not ask for clarification is the ultimate resistance myth (Estrich, 1987). The ultimate resistance myth is the social belief that true victims of sexual violence should provide ultimate resistance (Estrich, 1987), or at least appropriate resistance. Conversely, if the victim did *not* resist according to that standard or cannot provide evidence of resistance, the ultimate resistance myth allows the undermining inference that it is the victim's own fault.

This way of thinking is problematic because it shifts the responsibility and blame for sexual violence to the victim (e.g., Lonsway & Fitzgerald, 1994: 136). Furthermore, it shifts the burden of proof to the victim (Estrich, 1987). Also, this way of reasoning can present resistance as easy (Ehrlich, 2010: 269–270), while victims most likely were too scared of a further increase of violence, so that from the victim's perspective compliance or feigning compliance was the best available option (Ehrlich, 2002: 200–203). To add to the problematic nature of the myth, it has the status of 'common sense' reasoning that is pervasive in talk about sexual violence (MacLeod, 2016). This is also why it has been found so easy for cross-examiners in court to undermine rape victims' stories and present their attempts to resist as not enough (e.g., Ehrlich, 2002: 198–200).

In the data presented in this chapter, the resistance does not include cases of physical resistance, but the fact that in eleven instances children spontaneously give an account of misleading the alleged offender, suggests that there is a norm that makes such an account relevant. It is problematic that such a norm exists and that such young children apparently already orient to it, even without solicitation. Additionally, police officers do not necessarily accept the child's story, nor do they challenge the need to provide an account of resistance (cf. MacLeod, 2016). At the same time, not all vulnerable witnesses are able to pre-empt potential blame attributions. For example, Antaki et al. (2015b) demonstrate how witnesses with an intellectual disability often struggle to delete damaging implications when police officers probe inconsistencies. By contrast, we have seen one way in which children manage to pre-empt such damaging implications and blame attributions, despite the fact that children are subjected to the complex and alienating setting of the police interrogation. This can be seen as a display of interactional competence that is especially relevant given that the norm of resistance that is so pervasive in society.

Professional Reflection: The Dilemma of Working in the Best Interest of the Child in Sexual Abuse Cases and the Legal Process

Naomi Dessaur

Abstract

In my reflection on the findings of the chapter by Jol, Stommel and Spooren, I explicate some of the dilemmas of professionals in the legal field, even though they are committed to take the best interest of the child as a starting point for their work. One of the central dilemmas is how to safeguard the child to tell his/her own story, while also preventing the child from feeling pressured into taking legal steps and prosecuting a suspect. These dilemmatic situations may sometimes result in outcomes opposed to creating a safe, child-centered environment in which children can tell their story. In my profession, I have seen that children are smart enough to trick their abuser. This should however not be treated as a norm. I therefore want to make a plea for the claim that children are never guilty, whether they actively resist the abuse or not, and whatever the outcome of the legal process.

In article 3 of the UN Convention on the Rights of the Child (UNCRC, 1992) a reference is made to what is in 'the best interest of the child' when stating: "*in all actions concerning children, whether undertaken by public or private social welfare institutions, courts of law, administrative authorities or legislative bodies, the best interest of the child shall be a primary consideration*". In this contribution, I want to reflect on what counts as the best interest of the child, when the child is involved in the legal process, as this involvement can pose different types of dilemmas for the actual well-being of the child.

As an 18-year-old volunteer, I was confronted with sexual abuse of children at the Dutch Childline (Kindertelefoon). Most of the abuse was committed by an acquaintance or close relative of the family. At the Dutch Childline you are not supposed to act, give advice or find the truth; the story of the child is the most important and the story as it is told by the child counts as the child's truth. For me as a volunteer, this was sometimes frustrating (Berliner & Conte, 1995). We were not supposed to advise a child to go to the police or to stop the abuse. I felt that therefore we were not fully able to prevent abuse of other children who possibly could become victims as well. Looking back, 20 years later, on this period I realize that the Dutch Childline is one of the few places where a child can be open about his/her life without any kind of pressure for taking legal steps. This is worth its weight in gold. I always mention the example of the Dutch Childline to professionals for this very reason.

At twenty-two, I started to work as a case manager at the Dutch Child Protection Agency where children are guided in a volunteer framework. I worked with children who experienced sexual abuse and who were also in the middle of a legal process. During the eight years I worked at the Child Protection Agency, my opinion about the legal process, and what it means for children to be part of it, changed. I often felt a tension between what was supposedly in the best interest of the child and the importance of prosecuting a suspect. At the same time, it remains important to prosecute a suspect since that is the only way to stop the abuse.

As a trainer, I teach professionals how to conduct conversations with children about (suspicions of) sexual abuse and/or other forms of child neglect or abuse. During the training we discuss how there may be different interests at stake for the child when filing a police report and how this may pose dilemmas for the child. There is almost no 'right' choice. Of course the best interest of the child prevails, also at those times, but what does this mean if there are clear signs that the abuse is involving more children? There are no guarantees that the best interest of every single child can be served at those times and what sounds like an important goal to adhere to then seems so much harder to maintain. Consider for example the implications for children who are then asked to take up the role as a witness in an abuse case to strengthen the case against a suspect.

The Effects

To be a witness in an abuse case is often not without negative consequences for children (Vanoni, Lunemann, Kriek, Drost, & Smits van Waesberghe, 2013; Wijers & De Boer, 2010). The legal process is, as the chapter by Jol, Stommel & Spooren also shows, primarily about truth finding, collecting evidence and determining whether the sexual abuse did really happen. It is clear that on the one hand, we need such an objective and impartial process in an attempt to find the truth and to convict suspects. On the other hand there is the best interest of the child and whether that is served in those instances, for example when having to take part in multiple police interviews. I consider this to be another aspect of the paradox, which I cannot totally unravel, but which this chapter also illustrates.

In transcriptions of police interviews we often see that investigators start the interviews with a clear, and neutrally worded question, after which they encourage children to go on by verbal or non-verbal confirmation and by providing short summaries. Golden rules I teach professionals in my trainings are:

- the story of the child has to be taken seriously at all times;

- refrain from using leading questions as these provide suggestions as to which answer is preferred or considered 'best' or right';
- the child is master over her/his story.

I see comparisons between what I capture in these golden rules with what police inspectors who interview children do in practice, but I also often miss empathy and warmth in their method of interviewing (and questioning) children. I'll come back to this later.

It would be very good if we could find ways to convict suspects without the child, who has been the victim of the suspect, necessary play a role in the prosecution. Children can feel enormous pressure and guilt when a conviction is being made. To establish whether someone is guilty should maybe not depend on the story and experiences of the child. This is even more true when there is (some form of) loyalty with the abuser involved. This is something that is often the case when the abuse has taken place over a longer period of time and/or when there is (or has developed) a personal (family) bond. In those instances, feelings of guilt can even be stronger for the children involved.

The fear children can experience, long after the abuse has stopped must not be underestimated. Threats that abusers use with their victims are often unimaginably cruel and manipulative, which the following examples show. Abusers may say things like: "*I'll kill your mother if you tell anyone.*"; "*No one will believe you.*"; "*You wanted it yourself so you are also guilty.*"; "*I cut off your fathers ear.*"; "*If you tell anyone, I will harm your brother/sister.*" When fears like these play a role, talking to a police inspector or being involved in a legal process can be terrifying. In some instances, it might result in secondary traumatization and victimization. We speak of secondary traumatization when children are traumatized again by the legal process. In that case the post-traumatic stress reaction may deepen. This risk is especially high with victims of rape, violence or human trafficking. These children need recognition and support, while an interrogation, also in an informative way, can be felt like an attack on their personal credibility (Vanoni et al., 2013; Wijers & De Boer, 2010).

The way children are treated by the police, the influence of reactions of third parties or the attitude of the defense attorney can cause secondary victimization (Verwey-Jonker Institute, 2014: 17). The way children are treated may be considered too formal, or too much like there would be no difference between talking to children and talking to adults. The needs of the child victim might paradoxically as it seems, be overlooked when children are part of a legal process (Maas-de Waal, 2006).

It would be very good to avoid these risks for secondary traumatization and/or victimization. In Israel, there is a possibility to substitute the child in the legal process by a social worker, who will appear in court instead of the child (Morag, 1992). In cases of sexual abuse it is the social worker who talks with lawyers, police, prosecutor, defense and will also represent the child in court. This might be an interesting example to avoid the burden of telling your story time and again and to avoid involvement in the conviction. In the Israeli case, responsibility is removed from the child and transferred to an adult. However, in this Israeli format the social worker has to be trained to guarantee that the story he or she hears from the child in the first place is genuine and true. We still know very little about the ways in which social workers invite children to tell their story (but see van Nijnatten, 2013 for some of the characteristics of those talks in research conducted in the Netherlands).

Of course there is another side to this as well. Children can be relieved that the (sexual) abuse stops, that their story is heard, the abuser convicted. They may feel proud to be involved in this process. It can even restore their self-esteem. However, even though children might adapt well after such a traumatic experience, the lasting effects of having experienced (sexual)abuse should never be underestimated.

Offering Resistance

During many years of working with children of different ages, it has become clear that every child reacts differently to stressful and traumatic events. Not every child will actively and visibly resist sexual abuse. Some children will freeze (the so-called fight-or-flight response), dissociate or will do nothing, simply because they can't. In my opinion, doing nothing can also be a coping strategy and ensure the abuse to stop or even worse happening.

The question then also arises whether resisting or the lack of resistance should be taken as a decisive factor in determining whether sexual abuse has taken place. Can we talk about compliance or even some sort of compliance if it's based on inequality, which is always the case with sexual abuse of a minor? In the case of sexual abuse I think that a child can never be guilty, whether it actively and visibly resisted the abuse or not. As mentioned above, a child can be completely influenced, terrified by the manipulations, scared or indoctrinated and because of all those reasons, incapable to offer resistance.

Tricks

However, children are also capable to fool an abuser and use tricks. This shows how inventive and self-reliant children can be. I am still surprised how smart children sometimes are, in the circumstances, to deal with certain difficult situations and how they 'protect' themselves. To use the word protection in instances in which the sexual abuse does not stop is maybe an extraordinary term. Preventing or stopping violence and/or abuse are not the only ways to resist and protect oneself. Using tricks are a form of resistance as well, such as the trick that was mentioned in the chapter ('I pretended to sleep,' see fragment 4) or dissociation (an unconscious process, fleeing the situation), or using a pretend mode 'I needed to stay in school longer'. Similar to instances in which children freeze these can all be considered coping mechanism to prevent worse.

Recommendations

The strategies of deception discussed in the chapter by Jol and colleagues demonstrate the seriousness of the situation and the necessity for a coping strategy. The child had to dissociate or use a trick to survive. Resistance does not only show in spoken language.

An experience-expert and colleague who went through multiple forms of child abuse and sexual abuse, and is now working with victims of sexual abuse, said:

> I was raped by my father regularly between the age of five and eight. I very much wanted the sexual abuse to stop. I used tricks to make sure I would not utter a word since I was terrified, because my father threatened me with all sorts of terrible things. I literally had no words to tell what was happening. I was not able to give words to what happened with my body nor to convey the stress and fear I felt. How was I supposed to give words to the feeling of feeling completely insecure? At home I was not safe and my body and language also felt unsafe. I was terrified to speak up.

This girl was coping by keeping quiet and building up such muscle tension that she would not shiver and speak after the abuse. She might not have been able to tell her story to a police inspector and her abuser might not have been convicted. On the other side, the evidence was so overwhelming that even with her not being able to verbalize what she had experienced a conviction could have been the outcome. We may begin to see how warmth, support and empathy is an important factor and could have contributed to help this girl to be able to verbalize her experiences. After years of counseling and therapy, my colleague was able to tell her story and use it as an experience-expert.

In the fragments Jol, Stommel and Spooren present in their chapter, the police officers seem not to be warm or supportive. However in my opinion, whether or not they would be supportive probably not have hindered the interrogation. Abused children come from an unsafe environment. It is recommended to create a safe atmosphere before expecting children to tell their story, since telling your story to a stranger is quite unsafe anyway. Police officers may stay neutral, but this does not necessarily mean that they act in an 'unattached' manner. It is possible to be neutral and to be supportive at the same time. Examples I see in my work are giving a compliment, for instance, to express that it takes courage to tell this story. To explicitly state that a child can take the time it needs to say something (or not) or that the child is not to blame, whatever the outcome of the legal process.

I want to conclude by saying that my recommendations from the field are underlined by the policy recommendations by the Council of Europe for a child-friendly justice system and the Lanzarote Convention (2007).

The convention states helpful guidelines for states that are part of this Convention:

> Each Party shall take the necessary legislative or other measures to ensure that:
>
> a. interviews with the child take place without unjustified delay after the facts have been reported to the competent authorities;
> b. interviews with the child take place, where necessary, in premises designed or adapted for this purpose;
> c. interviews with the child are carried out by professionals trained for this purpose;
> d. the same persons, if possible and where appropriate, conduct all interviews with the child;
> e. the number of interviews is as limited as possible and in so far as strictly necessary for the purpose of criminal proceedings;
> f. the child may be accompanied by his or her legal representative or, where appropriate, an adult of his or her choice, unless a reasoned decision has been made to the contrary in respect of that person.

References

Antaki, C., Richardson, E., Stokoe, E., & Willott, S. (2015a). Police interviews with vulnerable people alleging sexual assault: Probing inconsistency and questioning conduct. *Journal of Sociolinguistics, 19*(3), 328–350.

Antaki, C., Richardson, E., Stokoe, E., & Willott, S. (2015b). Can people with intellectual disability resist implications of fault when police question their allegations of sexual assault and rape? *Intellectual and Developmental Disabilities, 53*(5), 346–357.

Antaki, C., Richardson, E., Stokoe, E., & Willott, S. (2015c). Dealing with the distress of people with intellectual disabilities reporting sexual assault and rape. *Discourse Studies, 17*(4), 415–432.

Berliner, L., & Conte, J. R. (1995). The effects of disclosure and intervention on sexual abused children. *Child Abuse and Neglect, 19*(3), 371–384.

Bolden, G. B., & Robinson, J. D. (2011). Soliciting accounts with *why*-interrogatives in conversation. *Journal of Communication, 61*(1), 94–119.

Childs, C., & Walsh, D. (2017). Self-disclosure and self-deprecating self-reference: Conversational practices of personalization in police interviews with children reporting alleged sexual offenses. *Journal of Pragmatics, 121*, 188–201.
Childs, C., & Walsh, D. (2018). Paradoxical invitations: Challenges in soliciting more information from child witnesses. *Research on Language and Social Interaction, 51*(4), 363–378.
Dekens, K., & van der Sleen, J. (2013). *Handleiding Het kind als getuige.* Amsterdam: Stapel & De Koning.
Ehrlich, S. (2002). (Re)contextualizing complainants' accounts of sexual assault. *Forensic Linguistics, 9*(2), 193–212.
Ehrlich, S. (2010). Rape victims: The discourse of rape trials. In M. Coulthard & A. Johnson (Eds.), *The Routledge handbook of forensic linguistics* (pp. 265–280). London and New York: Routledge.
Estrich, S. (1987). *Real rape.* Cambridge, MA: Harvard University Press.
Fogarty, K. (2010). *'Just say it in your own words': The social interactional nature of investigative interviews into child sexual abuse* (Unpublished thesis). University of Adelaide.
Fogarty, K., Augoustinos, M., & Kettler, L. (2013). Re-thinking rapport through the lens of progressivity in investigative interviews into child sexual abuse. *Discourse Studies, 15*(4), 395–420.
Frith, H., & Kitzinger, C. (1997). Talk about sexual miscommunication. *Women's Studies International Forum, 20*(4), 517–528.
Goodman, G. S. (1984). Children's testimony in historical perspective. *Journal of Social Issues, 40*(2), 9–31.
Hokwerda, Y. M., Veldman, T., de Graaf, L., & Rueb, C. (2015). *Minderjarige slachtoffers van seksueel misbruik in het strafproces. Een toetsing aan het internationale kinderrechtenkader.* Defence for Children.
Iversen, C. (2018). Filling in the gaps: Understanding beyond information in child social welfare interviews. *British Journal of Social Psychology, 58*(3), 550–568.
Jakobsen, K. K., Langballe, A., & Schultz, J. H. (2017). Trauma-exposed young victims: Possibilities and constraints for providing trauma support within the investigative interview. *Psychology, Crime and Law, 23*(5), 427–444.
Jefferson, G. (2004). Glossary of transcript symbols with an introduction. In G. Lerner (Ed.), *Conversation analysis: Studies from the first generation* (pp. 13–31). Amsterdam and Philadelphia: Benjamins.
Jol, G. (forthcoming). Children's unsolicited accounts and the illusion of neutral uptakes. In *Police interviews with child witnesses: Advice literature and actual talk (working title)* (Dissertation). LOT, Nijmegen.

Jol, G., & Stommel, W. (2016a). Resisting the legitimacy of the question: Self-evident answers to questions about sources of knowledge in police interviews with child witnesses. *International Journal of Legal Discourse, 1*(2), 345–374.
Jol, G., & Stommel, W. (2016b). Ethical considerations of secondary language use: What about informed consent? *Dutch Journal of Applied Linguistics, 5*(2), 180–195.
Kelly, L. (1988). *Surviving sexual violence.* Minneapolis: University of Minnesota Press.
Kitzinger, C., & Frith (1999). Just say no? The use of conversation analysis in developing a feminist perspective on sexual refusal. *Discourse & Society, 10*(3), 293–316.
Lamb, M. E., Orbach, Y., Hershkowitz, I., Esplin, P. W., & Horowitz, D. (2007). A structured forensic interview protocol improves the quality and informativeness of investigative interviews with children: A review of research using the NICHD Investigative Interview Protocol. *Child Abuse and Neglect, 31*(11–12), 1201–1231.
Lanzarote Convention. Art 35 of the CETS 201 (Lanzarote Convention) – *Protection of Children against Sexual Exploitation and Sexual Abuse*, 25.10.2007. https://www.coe.int/en/web/conventions/full-list/-/conventions/treaty/201.
Lonsway, K. A., & Fitzgerald, L. F. (1994). Rape myths: In review. *Psychology of Women Quarterly, 18*(1994), 133–164.
Luchjenbroers, J., & Aldridge, M. (2013). Do you kick a dog when it's down? Considering the use of children's video-recorded testimonies in court. In M. Freeman & F. Smith (Eds.), *Law and language, current legal issues* (Vol. 16, pp. 292–309). Oxford: Oxford University Press.
Maas-de Waal, C. J. (2006). *Voorzieningen voor slachtoffers van misdrijven. Gebruik, bereik en draagvlak.* The Hague: SCP.
MacLeod, N. (2016). "I thought I'd be safe there": Pre-empting blame in the talk of women reporting rape. *Journal of Pragmatics, 96*, 96–109.
Mandelbaum, J. (2013). Storytelling in conversation. In J. Sidnell & T. Stivers (Eds.), *The handbook of conversation analysis* (pp. 492–507). Chichester: Blackwell.
Ministerie van Veiligheid en Justitie. (2013). *Aanwijzing auditief en audiovisueel registreren van verhoren van aangevers, getuigen en verdachten.* http://wetten.overheid.nl/BWBR0032552/2013-01-01.
Ministry of Justice. (2011). *Achieving best evidence in criminal proceedings: Guidance for vulnerable or intimidated witnesses, including children.* London: Ministry of Justice.

Mondada, L. (2014). *Conventions for multimodal transcription.* https://franz.unibas.ch/fileadmin/franz/user_upload/redaktion/Mondada_conv_multimodality.pdf.
Morag, T. (1992). The law of evidence revision. In F. Lösel, D. Bender & T. Bliesener (Eds.), *Psychology and the law: International perspectives* (pp. 385–392). New York: De Gruyter.
National Rapporteur on Trafficing in Human Beings and Sexual Violence against Children. (2014). *On solid ground: Tackling sexual violence against children in the Netherlands.* The Hague: National Rapporteur.
Pomerantz, A. (1978). Compliment responses: Notes on the co-operation of multiple constraints. In J. Schenkein (Ed.), *Studies in the organization of conversational interaction* (pp. 79–112). New York: Academic Press.
Pomerantz, A. (1986). Extreme case formulations: A way of legitimizing claims. *Human Studies, 9*(2–3), 219–229.
Potter, J. (1996). *Representing reality: Discourse, rhetoric and social construction.* London: Sage.
Sacks, H. (1974). An analysis of the course of a joke's telling in conversation. In R. Bauman & J. Sherzer (Eds.), *Explorations in the ethnography of speaking* (pp. 337–353). Cambridge: Cambridge University Press.
Sacks, H. (1995). *Lectures on conversation.* Oxford: Blackwell.
Schegloff, E. (1997). "Narrative analysis" thirty years later. *Journal of Narrative and Life History, 7*(1–4), 97–106.
UNCR. (1992). *The United Nations Convention on the Rights of the Child.*
Van der Kruis, P. W. (2014). Het slachtofferdenken en het kind(on)vriendelijke studioverhoor. *Strafblad* (Mei), 150–156.
van Nijnatten, C. (2013). Downgrading as a counterstrategy: A case study in child welfare. *Child and Family Social Work, 18*, 139–148.
Vanoni, M., Lunemann, K. D., Kriek, F., Drost, L., & Smits van Waesberghe, E. (2013). *Meerwaarde integrale opvang en hulpverlening aan slachtoffers van seksueel geweld.* Amsterdam: Regioplan Beleidsonderzoek; Utrecht: Verwey Jonker Instituut.
Verwey Jonker instituut. (2014). *Maatregelen ter voorkoming van secundair en herhaald slachtofferschap.* Utrecht: Verwey-Jonker Instituut.
Wijers, M., & de Boer, M. (2010). *Een keer is genoeg: verkennend onderzoek naar secundaire victimisatie van slachtoffers als getuigen in het strafproces.* Utrecht: Marjan Wijers Research & Consultancy, WODC.
Woodhams, J., Hollin, C. R., Bull, R., & Cooke, C. (2012). Behavior displayed by female victims during rapes committed by lone and multiple perpetrators. *Psychology, Public Policy, and Law, 18*(3), 415–452.

6

Children's Competence and Wellbeing in Sensitive Research: When Video-Stimulated Accounts Lead to Dispute

Maryanne Theobald and Susan J. Danby

Professional Reflection by Gillian Busch

Introduction

Research studies increasingly recognize children as active participants deserving of social recognition and as key informants in matters that affect them. This view is driven by a child rights agenda (United Nations, 1989), 'competent child' paradigm (Hutchby & Moran-Ellis, 1998; Mackay, 1991; Speier, 1973) and Childhood Studies (Corsaro, 2017; Prout &

M. Theobald (✉) · S. J. Danby
School of Early Childhood and Inclusive Education, Queensland University of Technology (QUT), Brisbane, QLD, Australia
e-mail: m.theobald@qut.edu.au

S. J. Danby
e-mail: s.danby@qut.edu.au

J. Lamerichs et al. (eds.), *Children and Mental Health Talk*,
The Language of Mental Health,
https://doi.org/10.1007/978-3-030-28426-8_6

James, 1997), which suggest that children views and input are sought on a range of aspects regarding their everyday lives (for an overview see Tisdall, 2016). Such an approach shifts the research gaze from the child as an *object* of research to the child as an *active member* (Mason & Danby, 2011; Quennerstedt & Quennerstedt, 2014; Theobald, Danby, & Ailwood, 2011). Participatory approaches may promote better understanding of children's perspectives and enable child 'voice'; in research, however, when children exert their competence as research participants, the research encounter is unpredictable in nature, and matters to do with wellbeing may emerge.

The Unpredictable Nature of Research Encounters

The unpredictable nature of research means that research encounters with children, such as inviting children's perspectives in an interview, may not go according to the researcher's agenda, even with extensive preplanning on the part of the researcher. Guidelines may provide straight forward advice on how to undertake such an activity (see, e.g., Danby, 2017; Danby & Farrell, 2005). In reality, however, because the process of an interview is a mutually constructed and collaborative activity, there is scope for events to not go according to plan. For example, Danby, Ewing, and Thorpe (2011) showed how a novice researcher, who had undertaken multiple preplanning activities such as spending time in the classroom getting to know the children and undertaken practice interviews with young children, still found the interview process challenging. Reflecting on the interviews, the novice researcher commented that the interviews had produced limited conversation because the child participants had closed down topics and resisted answering the researcher-led questions. On closer examination of the interview data, though, the researcher realized that she had not made use of probing questions to extend the child's discussion and further found that having an activity or task to undertake at the same time as the interview promoted further discussion. When researching children's everyday lives, if something goes awry or is unexpected, researchers are expected to draw on their 'professional stock of knowledge' (Peräkylä & Vehvil*f*inen, 2003), by employing appropriate and skillful ethical principles *in situ*

(Graham, Powell, & Taylor, 2015). This might be particularly true when what might be described as 'sensitive' research is involved (Antaki, 2002).

Divulging Sensitive Issues

Children may employ a number of strategies when asked to divulge potentially 'sensitive' issues. For example, researching playground disputes, Theobald (2017) showed how three boys, aged 8 years, 'hijacked' the video-stimulated conversation by competently using interactional strategies to avert or side track the researcher's line of questioning. Their interactional strategies included interruptions, topic changes, non-verbal signals such as gaze, physical proximity and laughter to signal alignment with their peers and disaffiliation from the researcher. Similarly, Evang and Øverlien (2015) interviewed children about their experiences of family violence and found that children steered the researcher's questions away from topics that they did not wish to discuss. Asking children to discuss sensitive issues such as their experience of natural disasters (Bateman & Danby, 2013; Lamerichs, Alisic, & Schasfoort, 2018), risky behaviors (Daley, 2013) or matters to do with sexual orientation (Skelton, 2008) can also provide children with opportunities to disclose their feelings, enabling them to deal with and overcome trauma or upset. Such studies highlight their competence to comment on such sensitive issues. Conducting such research is not straightforward, however, it does provide children with opportunities to employ competence and agency as research participants. Exploring sensitive issues have ethical complexities for researchers, however, as they strive to 'do no harm' (Sharpe, 1997: 197) when conducting research.

Children's Wellbeing in Research Encounters

Researchers have responsibilities for ethical compliance to ensure children's wellbeing is regarded in research. Attention is given to the procedures of ethics with studies examining ongoing consent (Danby & Farrell, 2005; Mayne, Howitt, & Rennie, 2018) and increasingly the tensions between wellbeing, competence and children's participation are highlighted

(Skelton, 2008). These guidelines inform the kinds of topics investigated, the age of the children involved and how and where the research occurs (Daley, 2013; Farrell, 2016; Graham & Fitzgerald, 2010; Skelton, 2008). For the most part, children's participation in research is still routinely promoted as unproblematic for both researcher and child participant. Increasingly, however, studies are exploring the power differentials between adults and children (see Powell & Anderson, 2005); matters to do with how children's views are interpreted and responded to (see Dorner, 2014); the design of the questions that are asked of children (Danby et al., 2011; Lamerichs et al., 2018); the agency of children and what they bring to the researcher-participant interaction (Theobald, 2017). Although ethical guidelines work to ensure anonymity and protect vulnerable participants (Daley, 2013; Farrell, 2016), these guidelines do not always capture matters that arise regardless of planning for the process, researcher expertise and children's competence may be under-recognized or overruled. This matter is further explored in this chapter.

The Study

This chapter investigates a video-stimulated conversation among a small group of girls when accounting for their playground actions. The focus is on what happens when a dispute emerges. Data are from a video-ethnography that studied children's participation in a preparatory year classroom, colloquially referred to as 'prep,' with 24 children aged four to six years. The prep year is the first year of compulsory schooling in the Australian state of Queensland. The children attended an urban school in Southeast Queensland. The data collection process took place early in the school year as the classroom rules and procedures were being established. There were two data collection phases in the study. The first phase video-recorded the everyday experiences of the children interacting within the playground. The second phase used video-stimulated interviews where short fragments of the video-recorded episodes were shown to the participating children and the teacher (on separate occasions). They were asked to make comments on what is going on in the video fragments. These conversations, referred to as 'video stimulated accounts' (Pomerantz, 2005), were audio-recorded. This phase enabled children to take on a participatory role as they accounted for their experiences in the video-recorded play episodes and made points of interest.

The research encounter involved the researcher (first author) talking with a small group of girls aged 4–6 years as they watched a video-recording of themselves involved in a pretend game of 'school' in the playground. In this 'video-stimulated account' (Pomerantz, 2005; Theobald, 2012, 2017), the researcher's questions to the children about what was happening in the video clip lead to a dispute among the children. The dispute begins when one child initiates a complaint centered on an unresolved, and previously undisclosed, peer issue. The issue was that some children dominated the game by always wanting to be the 'teacher,' meaning that the others in the game were relegated to role of 'student' in the game, a role that did not have nearly the same authority as that of the self-assigned 'teacher.' This reflective activity of asking the children to talk about what was going on in the video creates a relational opportunity for some of the children to competently report on their own experiences, and they start to complain about one of the children involved in the play. The researcher faces the dilemma of how to resolve the dispute, one that she has inadvertently initiated, in a way that ensures the children's wellbeing, while acknowledging their competence in the video-stimulated account.

Analytical Approach

An ethnomethodological approach was taken using conversation analysis (Sacks, 1995; Sidnell & Stivers, 2012). Ethnomethodology studies the methods that people, including children, use to produce and make sense of social action. Conversation analysis employs fine-grained tools to uncover how social activities are produced and understood. As Garfinkel (1967) argued, there is a link between how people make sense of the world and their subsequent activities. Membership categorization analysis (MCA) also comes into play to examine the interactional tools that people use, and which are associated with particular categories (Fitzgerald, 2012; Sacks, 1972, 1995).

Using an ethnomethodological approach, video-stimulated accounts in this study are treated as interactional accomplishments in their own right and are not intended to test the recall of the participants or compare the account with the events that occurred. Accounts have been shown to be strategic conversational devices (Gill, 1998; Silverman, 1987; Theobald, 2012). Using an ethnomethodological lens, questions such as 'what work is the account doing?' and 'why that now?' guide analyses.

In using video-stimulated accounts, this study implements a method within ethnomethodological studies that has been relatively unused. Within this field, there are few studies that document the responses of participants who are viewing video sequences and none that include the views of young children. Pomerantz (2005) reports a study that collected video-recordings as well as audio-recorded video-stimulated comments of the medical interactions between doctor and adult patients. The research team found that the comments enabled them to focus on events in the interaction that otherwise might have been overlooked. The main focus of video-stimulated accounts is to tap into the participants' accounts for explanations of and concerns from the initial event, and it is not a recall method (Theobald, 2017). Video-stimulated accounts provide a chance for children to provide their standpoint and inform data analysis and showed the children's social worlds as multifaceted (Theobald, 2012). In sum, the '*interpretations*, *aims* and *concerns* to which the participants may have oriented' (Pomerantz, 2005: 93, emphasis in original) can be exposed.

The video-stimulated accounts came from an extended sequence of interaction. Extended sequences provide analysts opportunities to understand how talk and interaction are instigated and unfold (Psathas, 1992). The next section introduces fragments of this extended conversation of approximately 15 minutes, between the researcher and the children who were involved in watching a video recording of themselves playing a pretend game of school.

First, the original interaction captured on video (a game of school) is described. Second, seven transcribed accounts of the video-stimulated conversation are presented for analysis. Transcription methods followed typical CA protocols using the Jefferson (2004) technique (see Appendix 1). This transcription method highlights the interactional details of the talk and interaction such as intonation, overlap, pauses and volume. These features provide analysts with clues into how the members are interpreting and responding to each other in the interaction. Pseudonyms are used for all names in the transcript.

Setting the Scene: A Game of School

In the playground, the researcher previously had observed and video-recorded six girls, Becky, Maddy, Cindy, Georgia, Ella and Macy, who were playing a pretend game of school. Each girl had taken a pretend role by drawing on the categories of student and teacher. Maddy, Cindy and Becky were teachers and the others played the role of students in the school. Playing the role of a 'student' required Georgia, Ella and Macy to follow the instructions and perform the duties outlined by the 'teachers'. The next day, the researcher asked the group of girls to watch and comment on the play episode in a video-stimulated account. At the beginning of the session, the researcher asked, 'what's going on there,' and the girls reported that a game of school was the activity being played. The conversation is picked up when the researcher comments on a disparity in how the game is reported and the lack of display of enjoyment.

Account 1: Accounting for unhappy faces in the game

```
R'cher:     'Cause I noticed di-you said it was fun to play the game
            tch but Ma-Ella and Macy and Georgia (0.4) at one stage you
            didn't have very happy fa:ces?
            (0.5)
            were you feeling?- how were you feeling then.
            (1.2)
R'cher:     Georgia?
Georgia:    Well (0.4) um t sometimes we fi:ghted because Maddy always
            be'ed the teacher because um Becky fighted becaused Mad-
            .hhbecause she ne:ver getted to be the teacher because Ma-
            was always the teacher and Cindy was always the teacher.
R'cher:     Ah,
Maddy:      Well then I let her be the teacher.
R'cher:     [An oh    ]
Macy:       [And we n]ever be the teacher.
```

This account starts with the researcher using a formulation as she comments on how the disparity between the girls reports of what has come so far, their reports of feeling happy playing the game of school and their unhappy faces (lines 1–5). In so doing, however, the researcher steers the agenda or what Heritage and Watson (1979) describe as '"fix" ...(the) topic' (p. 149). As will be shown, this statement holds the girls accountable for their actions and is integral in directing the agenda for the remaining interview.

The pauses in the talk (lines 6) demonstrate a potential trouble in the interaction. The researcher selects Georgia to talk (line 7). Georgia hesitantly explains that Maddy is always the teacher. Her account starts by nominating that they all fought with Maddy, 'we fi:ghted because Maddy always be'ed the teacher' (lines 8–9). She then nominates Becky, who is not present at the interview, as the one who fights about being the teacher. Although initially Georgia named Maddy as always being the teacher, she later also includes Cindy (line 11), attempting to shift the course of the upset.

The shift from 'we' to naming Becky enables Georgia to competently nominate an absent party. This aversion may be the recognition that a dispute is not seen favorably by adults and particularly so by teachers. Georgia acts as an observer and reports Becky, the absent party, as being responsible for making complaints. Georgia instigates a complaint about Maddy on behalf of a third party not present. Similar to the 'he said-she said' scenarios identified by Goodwin (1990: 194), the provocation begins with relaying what one member accused another of in their absence.

Maddy treats Georgia's turn as a complaint and her next turn is a justification of her actions for a shared solution, 'Well then I let her be the teacher' (line 1). At the very beginning of the account, Maddy was named the owner of the idea for the game, a powerful position as the owner has control of the interactional decisions that follow. Another member, Macy, however, does not let this stand and further adds, 'And we never be the teacher' (line 15), effectively ignoring Maddy's comment. As interviewer, the researcher too lets this stand and continues with questioning about sad faces.

Account 2: 'So why did you keep playing if you were sad'

R'cher: So why did you [keep playing] (to Georgia)
Maddy: [jus-]
R'cher: if you were sad playing the game,
(1.3) ((sound from Ella))
R'cher: Ella?
Ella: Um (0.5) .hhnobody (0.5) if you weren't (any)
show anybody's fa:ce and some'dy might come and
help you up?
Maddy: Umm and (0.4) [we took them,]
R'cher: [In the ga:me?]A:h,so you were
showing a sad face [in the game but=]
Ella: [mmm.]
R'cher: =you weren't really sad.
(0.5)
Georgia: °Mhm°
R'cher: Is that what was happening Georgia?
(0.8)
Georgia: mm-[muh]
R'cher: [Oh wou]-what were you sad- (0.2) why did you
have a sad face?
(0.5)
Georgia: We:ll (0.5)um (0.6) we:ll (0.6).mhht we didn't-we
all er: (0.6)we-we didn't-we didn't really cr:y
when our mums (0.5)and dads left.
(1.2)
R'cher: N:o?
(0.6)
Georgia: Because (0.3) um (0.3)t- (0.7) she's talking
about um (0.7) it's (0.6) she's saying i-it's
bete::nding.
R'cher: It w's pretending. ah no So you were pretending
in the game, (0.3)mmm But-but were you happy to
pla:y the game? or were you-[were you wanting to]
go somewhere else?
Georgia: [mmmaa]
(0.5)
Georgia: Ah [we want (0.3) to]
R'cher: ['cause Ella an' Macy]an' Mad-an' you didn't
look very happy;
(1.7)
Georgia: Ye:ah because um (0.5) .hhh because <Maddy didn't
really let us play someting?>
R'cher: You wanted to be the teacher you said before.
Georgia: No well we-we wanted to play >something else and
Maddy said we can't play a:nything else<

In this account, the researcher's next question asks more about the girls' playing of the game. She asks Georgia, 'So why did you keep playing if you were sad playing the game.' Maddy's talk overlaps with the researcher's talk, providing what might be some kind of objection (line 24). After the researcher's question, there is a 1.3-second gap. Ella makes a sound and the researcher selects her to respond. Ella's explanation suggests the action of being sad was part of the pretense of playing the game (28–30) At this point, Georgia interjects with quiet 'mhm' sound, perhaps suggesting some resistance against this account. This is a crucial point in the video-stimulated interaction. Georgia could have agreed with Ella's explanation, but Georgia's next turns (lines 44–52) explicitly reveal the different frames of reference the girls are operating in, pretend versus real.

As the researcher continues to pursue the notion of being happy (lines 53–56), a complaint about Maddy emerges from Georgia (64–68). Georgia's complaint moves from the pretend frame to the actual framing of the activity. A new social order is underway, one that has moved from an account of pretend crying children to a real frame where Georgia points out, 'Maddy didn't really let us play someting?' (line 68). Provided with the conversational space by the researcher to expand on the game play, Georgia presents herself as a competent informant by offering a complaint to do with the real frame. The complaint sequence continues and escalates as the conversation progresses.

Account 3: 'We're getting bored of it'

```
Georgia:   =we al:ways play tha:t ga:me a:nd, and um Macy and me and
           E:lla wanted to >play somewhere different because we
           always play that game and we're getting bo:red
           [of it<.     ]
R'cher:    [so why didju] sta:y
           (1.2)
Georgia:   We:ll (0.5) tch (0.3) well she: (0.5) well Maddy didn't
           want us to g:o.
R'cher:    A:h.
Maddy:     We did-I didn't want them to go cos I don't want them to
           go ho:me.
R'cher:    O:h. So whose decision was it to sta:y then,
           (0.5) ((Ella puts hand up))
R'cher:    Ella?
Ella:      Um becau:se they [al-   ]
Maddy:                      [No Ma]ddy's (0.2) say Maddy's. please?
```

```
Ella:       You al:ways play with us=
Maddy:      [yeh-]
Ella:       [=and] we never playing with [(someone-)]
Maddy:                                   [N:O       ] (0.5) mm (0.6)
            it's not like that. She didn't mean-she didn't say tha:t.
Ella:       Yo:u al:ways play with us gu::ys,
Maddy:      No she didn't say that billy.
R'cher:     Well what well what are you trying to say Ella?
Ella:       Maddy and Cindy always plays with me and Macy and
            Georgia.
R'cher:     A:[h.]
Maddy:        [No] we do:n't.
R'cher:     And how do you feel about that?
Ella:       Becos they always-
Maddy:      Oka:y I'm not going to listen if you're going to be like
            this Ella,=
Ella:       =>I don't kno:w, I forgot [(all) I think-<]
R'cher:                               [How do you     ] fe:el about
            that Ella?
Ella:       I don't kno:w. I forgo:t.
R'cher:     A:h. (1.2) [mmmhh]
Ella:                  [.hhh ] [hh. ((sighs))          ]
Georgia:                       [And an' I never get to play] with
            Brigid because (0.2) she's actually my really best (0.3)
            friend and I feel sad about it-
```

As a complaint sequence is launched by Georgia (line 83), a history of discontent among the girls is evidenced with the descriptor of *always* locating the trouble source, '=we al:ways play tha:t ga:me' (line 85). Georgia supports her turn with an explanation to justify her complaint, presenting herself as a credible and competent participant.

The researcher orients to Georgia as a competent participant by inviting her to further account for her actions of playing the game, despite her lack of enjoyment of that game. Georgia's response makes relevant a rule nominated by the girls earlier: not going away. As a student in the game of school, Georgia is categorically bound to play the role of a student and to obey the instructions of the teacher in the game. However, if this comment is considered as real and not in the pretense frame, it refers to a code of conduct of how to be a friend. Georgia's explanation suggests that, as a member of the social group, she is morally obligated to follow the rules of the game and show alliance to the code of conduct.

When asked about who makes the decisions, Ella now complains about Maddy always playing with them. The use of an indexical expression (Heritage, 1984) in Maddy's response, it is not like 'tha:t' (line 103), is unclear to an outsider but is presented to Ella as one that she would understand as an insider. Maddy here poses some doubt as to Ella's competence, suggesting that Ella has misunderstood the researcher's question.

The girls carry on the conversation between themselves. The researcher is now an observer to their interaction. Maddy's naming of Ella as a *billy*, saying 'No she didn't say that billy.' (line 105), suggests a characterization of Ella as a *silly billy*. In so doing, Maddy calls into question Ella's competence and explicitly portrays her as someone whose opinion should not be counted on, as she is *not* a competent member. The 'overall competence of one who would produce that talk' could be in doubt (Goodwin & Goodwin, 1987: 210).

This matter has relational consequences. The girls have taken a number of turns to voice their complaints and accusations, highlighting the delicate interactional work being conducted in this interaction. Ella's alignment with Georgia and Macy has the potential to divide the group. Such a matter is not something that can be launched into lightly but rather one built over turns. Maddy cuts Ella's turn, telling her, 'Oka:y I'm not going to listen if you're going to be like this Ella,=' (lines 113–114). Maddy has predicted the trajectory of Ella's talk and uses what Church (2016) describes as a 'conditional threat.' This threat competently brings attention to Ella's telling and is possibly a pre-sequence to future courses of action of retelling.

Maddy's response to Ella's complaint moves the interaction forward to a multiparty dispute (Maynard, 1986). A dispute occurs in three parts, first turn is one child's action or talk, second another child responds negatively to first child's action or talk and third, the first child subsequently resists the complaint or control over their actions (Antaki, 1994; Cromdal, 2004; Danby & Theobald, 2012; Maynard, 1985a). Identified by Heritage and Watson (1979) as an upshot, this move by Maddy works to gag Ella. Ella immediately says, '=>I don't kno:w, I forgot (all) I think-<' (line 115). The use of *I don't know* can be used to bring the line of questioning to a close as Hutchby's (2002) study of talk in child counseling shows. If Ella continues with her accusation, she is displaying an affiliation to Georgia and Macy in front of Maddy, and her current relationship with Maddy is uncertain. The others are noticeably silent in this exchange.

Ella's turn, 'I don't know' is used as a justification for abandoning her complaint, which provides a momentary halt to the emerging dispute.

In so doing, Ella is orienting to the rules of play of 'not going away' and related moral obligations as a member of the peer group. Georgia's discussion about playing with her 'best' friend, Brigid, employs historical and local understandings as justifications. This dialogue is embedded with historical references that refer to past disputes and social orders, drawing on obligations as a member of the peer culture (to play with her 'best' friend).

Account 4: 'Stop talking about me'

```
R'cher:     So why is Maddy the boss of you where there's
            (0.8) places to pla:y?
Ella:       No only the teachers are the boss of this whole
            school. Umm the whole teachers.
Georgia:    Um actually [the principal         ]
R'cher:                 [so wh-                ]
Maddy:                  [No the principal is.]
R'cher:     so who makes the decisions about where you pla:y
            though?
Gerogia:    [The principals.]
Maddy:      [The principals.]
R'cher:     What about when you're outside.
Georgia:    [Uh              ]
Ella:       [The principal.  ]
R'cher:     [If you wanned to] go somewhere else couldn't
            you decide t[o go somewhere else?]
Georgia:                [A n d   t h e n   u m] (0.3) w'll I
            [rea:lly wa:nt-]
Maddy:      [Stop  ta:lking] about me:.
            (0.4)
Georgia:    < I re:ally, re:ally want to jis play 'iv a
            different kind of friend¿ > .hhh I really wanna
            play wiv [(0.5) Sawy-            ]
Maddy:               [STOP talking about me,]
Georgia:    Sawyer
Maddy:      I'm getting upset.
Georgia:    An an I never get to play with Sawyer.
R'cher:     Oh.
Ella:       And I never get to play with uh Sawyer as well.
```

Picking up the interaction a few moments later, the researcher instigates a line of the questioning about the social order of the group, naming Maddy as the 'boss' (line 131). Ella disagrees and says, 'Umm the whole teachers' (line 134). Ella's comment may refer to the real teachers, not the pretend game. Using membership categorization devices (Sacks, 1972), the girls collaboratively and competently reject the researcher's suggestion of Maddy as the boss, by constructing the notion of 'boss' as the principal from the category group and institution, school. Here, we see the shift from a suggested boss of a pretend game, Maddy, to the real boss of the school, the principal.

In the next turn, the researcher appears to be displaying an epistemic standpoint about the interaction being discussed (see Antaki, 2002). The question, 'If you wanted to go somewhere else couldn't you decide to go somewhere else?' (line 145), is posed as a negative interrogative (Heritage, 2002) and suggests that the girls could not play anywhere else. This question, directed to Georgia and Ella, but not Maddy, separates the group and works to exclude Maddy. It also indicates to Maddy that the researcher is aligned with the perspectives of the other girls. Maddy picks up on this marginalization in her turn. She overlaps with Georgia's turn and, before any indication of the trajectory of Georgia's turn, says, 'Stop ta:lking about me:' (line 149). At that point, no one was talking about her. Maddy's directive may be responding to the girls' earlier talk about playing the game. Several times in the prior talk, her name is associated with negative implications and unequivocal complaints. It might act as an interactional warning to Georgia and the others that they are not following their moral obligations as members of the group. In the case of the latter, it is evidence that a code of conduct is at work in the interactional matters at hand here. Maddy's turn here can be viewed as a warning to the girls to follow this code.

Georgia responds by categorizing Maddy as a certain kind of friend, perhaps one that doesn't follow the suggested code of conduct. Georgia brings into play the moral obligations of the membership category of a friend, seen as an attempt to weaken Maddy's social status in the group. Georgia continues to tell about her desire to play with a 'different kind of friend' (line 152). This statement categorizes Maddy as one kind of friend, and Sawyer as another kind of friend. As both Georgia and Ella name Sawyer as someone with whom they would like to play, they competently make public their alignment and further marginalize Maddy's social position.

Account 5: 'I'm getting upset'

```
Maddy:     [We:ll-jus STOP              ] [talking-  ]
Macy:      [An I never get to play with]
R'cher:                                   [Wel-how do] what
           do you think Maddy?
Maddy:     I just don't want them to talk about me anymore
           'cause ~[it's getting me up-]~
R'cher:            [Well they're just t]alking about
           playing with Sawyer; they're not really talking
           about you are they?
Maddy:     Well they are because they're saying I don't get
           to play with um Sawyer and ~they-that means they
           are talking about me so I'm getting upset.~
           (0.9)
R'cher:    Ah? Why are you getting upset?
           (0.6)
Maddy:     Becos they're just being ~me:an (0.2) about me,~
           (0.9)
R'cher:    What are they-how are they being mean?
Maddy:     'Cos they're saying (1.2) um (3.5)
           well I don't know rea:lly what they're saying
           but they're just being mean about me.
R'cher:    Oh, (.) is that-is that what's happening?
```

As the account continues, Maddy portrays herself as a victim as she tells of her feelings of upset, using a tremulous voice. Addressing the other girls in the third person (line 164) is strategic, because it positions the other members of the interaction as an overhearing audience (see Heritage, 1985). Telling can be seen as a strategy to seek alignments from others (Maynard, 1985b, 1986; Theobald & Danby, 2017). Here, Maddy attempts to defend her position to the researcher. Maddy, the accused in the previous accounts, now narrates feelings of *getting upset* (line 165) and positions herself as the innocent party. There is a crossing here of who is now the offender and who is the offended (Goodwin, 1990). In so doing, Maddy attempts to recast herself.

The girls make known Maddy's reduced status in the group by reporting that they would rather play with others. Maddy makes explicit the particular moral order of the group at play, by drawing on previously reported obligations of the group (not shown here), not to talk about each other.

As the account continues, the researcher manages Maddy's claims of upset by further questioning her. In so doing, the researcher acknowledges her feelings and presents an opportunity for Maddy to give her version of events. A similar technique was observed by Danby and Theobald

(2012) in their study of a teacher managing two children's accounts of a playground dispute. Similar to the teacher in Danby and Theobald's (2012) study, the researcher, working in the category of teacher, shows respect to Maddy's competence and authority by asking her to further account for how she is feeling. Maddy takes this opportunity to respond and, in so doing, the affective display of upset seems to lessen, as noted by the more even voice as she takes her turn. The researcher here, acting in the membership category of teacher, is successful in momentarily disrupting the ongoing dispute exchange between the children.

Account 6: 'Well, now I'm upset'

```
Maddy:      'Cause they're saying (1.2) um (3.5) well I
            don't know rea:lly what they're saying but
            they're just being mean about me.
            Oh, (.) is that-is that what's happening?
R'cher:     (0.6)
Georgia:    Not re:ally.
R'cher:     N[o.]
Maddy:       [N:]o you're making me mean now.
R'cher:     Not really, [Georgia-Georgia think-]
Maddy:                  [You're making me upset]
R'cher:     Georgia is saying that she doesn't think she's
            rea:lly being mean, (1.3) [she's just] trying to
Maddy:                                [an I      ]
R'cher:     tell (0.7) me where she'd like to play (0.3)
            >who she'd like to play with< Is that right
            Georgia?
            (0.5)
Maddy:      I just like playing school=
R'cher:     You like to play school do you?
Maddy:      =with [my friend.   ]
R'cher:           [Do the other-]Do you like to play school
            then?
Georgia:          [No::::o.     ]
Ella:             [No::::o.     ]
Macy:             [No::::o.     ]
Georgia:    [I like to-]
Maddy:      [Well now  ] well now I'm ups:et.
Georgia:    I do like to play scho:ol (0.2) if I ne:ver play
            scho:ol.
Maddy:      but we never play school now I changed my mind I
            [never want to be the boss]
R'cher:     [°oh-so-°                 ]
            (3.0)
Maddy:      Stop giving me (hop)
            (2.8)
```

The dispute further intensifies in this account, as Maddy reframes her account to now portray the others as perpetrators. By explicitly identifying their action, 'being mean' (line 180), she categorizes Georgia, Ella and Macy as bullies. Maddy is doing what Maynard (1986) described as 'political' work here by soliciting support from a powerful third party, in this case the adult. *Meanness* is a tellable offense and one that typically stirs adults into action.

Maddy's affective state is evident in her mounting claims to being upset. She suggests that the comments that have been made are portraying her in a bad light, 'making me mean' (line 185), and she proposes a case of mistaken identity. There is a pronoun shift to '*you're* making me upset' (line 187), which competently attributes the blame to others. As the complaints continue, Maddy claims, 'Well now well now I'm ups:et' (line 204), the elongated and stressed talk also displaying her affected state. This narration about her escalation of feelings is achieved by its sequential placing: It comes directly after Georgia, Ella and Macy express, explicitly and strongly, their dislike of playing the game of school. In this way, Maddy's narrative sequence performs the social action of constructing a particular version of events that has to do with what Edwards (1999) described as blame and responsibility.

The narrative sequence affords Georgia, Ella and Macy the interactional space in which to back down from telling. Maddy's reported change of state works as a warning, and as a justification for her accusatory position and her view that she is offended, displays her competence achieving the upper hand in the dispute. The girls' complaint about Maddy has now been engineered by Maddy.

Maddy draws strategically on moral obligations from the membership category of classmates that were earlier articulated: that friends do not upset one another. This is an attempt to strengthen her social status in the group and solicit support from the other members. Similarly, in her Swedish study of the interactions of preadolescent girls in a playground, Evaldsson (2007) described talking about someone responsible for the trouble in her presence as a salient feature of the girls' talk. Evaldsson found that some members employed a taken-for-granted moral order that friends should not fight in order to advance their social status in the group.

It appears that Maddy's portrayal of herself as the victim has been effective for her social agenda. Georgia's next turn is a repair of a possible breach of moral order, 'I do like to play scho:ol (0.2) if I ne:ver play scho:ol' (lines 205–206). In this turn, Georgia gives an account for her not liking school—they play it too much. Georgia here competently diffuses the situation and attempts to appease Maddy, who responds now with a different line of defense. She addresses and makes explicit what she infers is the cause of the interactional trouble, 'but we never play school now I changed my mind I never want to be the boss' (lines 207–208). Maddy demonstrates to Georgia, Ella and Macy a willingness to act according to their particular code of conduct. The shared understanding made obvious here implies a previous history around this issue of being the boss.

Account 7: 'What do you think would be fair?'

```
R'cher:    So what do you think would be [fair? =]
Maddy:                                   [Can we] watch a
           bit more?
Georgia:   [Um       ]
R'cher:    [=in prep?]
           (1.0)
Georgia:   We:ll this what'd be fa:ir (.) we just take
           turns to playing each [<one of the ga:mes?> ].
Macy:                            [°(and we can play)°  ]
Georgia:   So first we have Maddy's game first like so we
           play school first then we play my game then we
           play .hhhElla's game then we play Macy's game
           and then we play Cindy's game.
R'cher:    Oh what did you say Macy?
Macy:      Uh
R'cher:    What did you just say? I didn't hear you.
Macy:      You have to be [kind to other people?   ]
Maddy:                    [Can we watch a bit more?]
R'cher:    You have to be kind to other people.
```

In the final account, the researcher here takes on the membership category and professional stock of knowledge associated with that of a teacher. In so doing, she orients to the typical rules of behavior in a classroom and attempts to restore a particular social order in the group. Promoting fairness is part of the learning outcome, *wellbeing*, outlined in the curriculum documents that support Australian early years settings (Department of Education, Employment & Workforce Relations [DEEWR], 2009).

Georgia responds to the researcher's question by detailing an elaborate plan for taking turns while they play (lines 222–225). In so doing, she indicates an alignment to a classroom order of wellbeing and fairness. Macy suggests being kind, which also invokes moral obligations of a classroom member and friend, responding to the category of teacher in play. Maddy's interruptions, suggesting they watch more of the video recording, may be a way of diverting further complaints about the sensitive issue to do with the playground game.

Discussion

Analyses revealed the competence of the children when asked to divulge and account for sensitive issues. Accounts do interactional work (Silverman, 1987). At the beginning of the interaction, the girls' responses portrayed an epistemic position, a claim to knowledge (O'Reilly, Lester, & Muskett, 2016), that indicated to the researcher that there was more to be told. The researcher's question design, use of formulations and continued pursuit of a topic jointly constructed the video-stimulated account and subsequent dispute. These actions offered some of the girls an interactional space to introduce their own relational agendas, which involved making complaints about one member of the peer group.

Making a complaint with an adult present was strategic. The complaint itself was an action constructed with others, and in front of others, with potential consequences for the complainants and the defendant. For example, talking about the offender in her presence meant in turn that the offender, the subject of the talk, could present a counter view or amend the situation. Through their inferences to rules, the girls attempted social exclusion and alignment with others and enforced their own social position. This resulted in a dispute arising and one of the girls, Maddy, claiming upset, a state that compromises feelings of wellbeing.

Children's disputes have implications for children's mental health and wellbeing and for researchers investigating children's these sensitive issues. Although Maddy did not actually cry, she did narrate a highly emotional state of upset, a potential concern for the researcher. Thus, the situation posed an ethical dilemma for the researcher, who worked between two membership categories, that of a researcher and teacher. On the one hand, the researcher was interested to uncover more about the interactional trouble instigated, while still ensuring ethical practice in research. On the other hand, the researcher was also a teacher, who in this membership category has a duty of care with an interest in promoting positive relationships. As an experienced teacher, the researcher would have experience in routinely managing disputes. In this interaction, she was able to draw upon her pedagogic expertise and her 'professional stock of knowledge' (Peräkylä & Vehvilƒinen, 2003) of a teacher to acknowledge Maddy's upset while still enabling the other girls' interactional space to share their feelings. In the end, however, the membership category of teacher overruled the researcher's questioning, and she attempted to restore the social order of the classroom. Following ethical procedures associated with the project, the researcher also discussed with the teacher the upset that Maddy claimed and the possible support that the teacher might later provide.

Video-stimulated accounts provide children with an opportunity to discuss their play interactions, therefore acknowledging their competence in managing their relationships and manipulating social situations. There is an 'interdependency between children's 'voice' and their sociocultural environments' (Horgan, 2017: 247). Accounts of friendship, moral obligations and feelings of wellbeing arise after watching the play episode and these have consequences for their future relationships.

With more and more studies involving children as competent participants, it is likely that researchers will seek strategies for how to manage research encounters in ways that are ethical and sensitive to children's wellbeing. We provide three suggestions to support children's wellbeing in research encounters, while still recognizing their competence. First, providing opportunities for children to provide an account and have an opportunity to respond is important. This positions children to provide their views and be involved in analyzing their everyday lives. The researcher, however, should be aware of the complexities and consequences of such positioning, as identified by the growing number of studies (see Farrell, 2016; Horgan, 2017). Second, careful attention should be given to the researcher stance and question design. As shown here, question design in research shapes ongoing talk and subsequent interactional conditions.

Third, efforts should be undertaken to understand the symbiotic relationship between gaining children's perspectives and social environments. As shown, what is discussed has immediate and future implications for relationships and children's ultimate wellbeing. Fourth, this episode highlighted the importance for researchers to be well prepared for providing external and follow up support to participants. Such support might involve, for example, reference to teachers and parents, while still respecting the confidentiality of children's accounts.

This chapter has provided an illustration of how a research encounter, where children were invited to be competent informants of matters that affect their own lives, can unfold. Using an ethnomethodological lens and turn-by-turn conversation analysis, findings highlighted the children's orientation toward the contestation of their social rights. Meanwhile, the researcher was faced with a dilemma to do with respecting children's competence and agency, pursuing answers or ensuring wellbeing. It is hoped that the findings presented here will provoke further discussion to inform researchers who seek to conduct sensitive research.

Professional Reflection

Gillian Busch

Abstract

In this research encounter, I was struck by how the researcher managed the multiple membership categories to which she belonged and the obligations attributed to each category. I can see a number of strategies that the researcher uses that might support me in my research with children, such as acknowledging the feelings of the children or reading the non-verbal cues proffered by the children as they engage with each other and with the researcher. Here the researcher, perhaps drawing on her knowledge and obligations as a teacher, recognizes that the class teacher needs to be informed about the upset claimed by the child during the interview. This brings to the fore the link to professional ethics as outlined in the Early

Childhood Australia (ECA) *Code of Ethics*, which foregrounds the importance of negotiating 'children's participation in research, by taking into account their safety' (ECA, 2016).

Beginning to write a reflection in response to analysis of rich data required that I gain familiarity with both the data and the analysis provided in the chapter. So, in approaching this task my focus is on what I can learn from other researchers who, like me, are deeply interested in finding out about children's perspectives on matters of importance to them.

As both a teacher of young children and researcher of and with children, I was struck by how the researcher managed the multiple membership categories to which she belonged and the obligations attributed to each category. Although all researchers engage in thoughtful planning, which includes submission of ethics' approvals, the reality of doing the research, particularly with young children, is often unpredictable in nature.

One consideration when researching ethically is to ensure the wellbeing of the children. In this research encounter, I can see a number of strategies that the researcher uses that might support me in my research with children. This includes acknowledging the feelings of the children, reading the non-verbal cues proffered by the children as they engage with each other and with the researcher and also providing acknowledgements such as 'ah' or 'oh' that seem to encourage the children to continue with their talk about how they feel and why they feel that way. Although confidentiality is important in research, here the researcher, perhaps drawing on her knowledge and obligations as a teacher, recognizes that the class teacher needs to be informed about the upset claimed by the child during the interview. For me, this brings to the fore the link to professional ethics as outlined in the Early Childhood Australia (ECA) *Code of Ethics*, which foregrounds the importance of negotiating 'children's participation in research, by taking into account their safety' (ECA, 2016). In some ways, being a researcher and a teacher are not discrete undertakings, rather, each category carries with it obligations that collectively inform how I will approach my research with children.

Reflecting on the transcripts included in this chapter, it is apparent that the researcher has immense familiarity with the video data the children were asked to discuss, and while it is not evident in the transcripts, it is apparent that the researcher's choice of video data to discuss with the children was also thoughtful. Thinking about this, I reflect on the way in which a conversation analytic approach urges researchers to have intimate familiarity with their data, and I consider my own work and the familiarity I have with data used for analysis. When using video-stimulated accounts with children, it seems that this familiarity with data is perhaps especially important. This is possibly because the researchers need to be able to select fragments and ask questions that enable the co-construction of accounts by the children and the interviewer. Familiarity with their data is also important to enable the researcher to construct formulations of what occurred and be able to recognize the agendas to which the members refer—both the local agendas (the unfolding disputes) and the earlier agendas referred to by the children. This capability would not be possible without that intimate familiarity with the data. Acknowledging that this familiarity is central to the production of video-stimulated accounts, the researcher commented that the video-stimulated conversations occurred the day following the recording. The closeness of the original recording time and children's opportunity to reflect seem to align with the methodology, but it does problematize how, as a researcher, I can decide on fragments to use with children and also become familiar with the data in a very short period of time. It might mean that this kind of work is done in consultation with a team of researchers—but of course many other implications might unfold if engaging in the process.

Following further examination of how the researcher managed the interaction with the children, I identified a number of features or strategies used by the researcher. Observations of how these interactional tools supported the children to co-construct video-stimulated accounts (Pomerantz, 2005) is now discussed.

First, the researcher used formulations (Sacks, 1995) of what happened in the video recording or what was said in a previous turn. For example, in account one, the researcher provides a formulation of a noticing of a mismatch between the observable emotions of the girls and what they indicate is happening. In posing the formulation, the researcher makes explicit what was being said or inferred by the children and prompts the children to account for why things occurred. So, in approaching the task of engaging in video-stimulated accounts, as a researcher, it is important that I understand how formulations are used by researchers and that I am aware how such formulations may steer the agenda or the topic rather than follow the direction decided by the children. So, again, researching with children remains tricky as attempts are made to find out about their perspectives and supporting them to accomplish this task.

Second, in a number of accounts, the researcher explicitly requests clarification about what the children were talking about and why they acted as they did, which elicits an extended complaint by some of the members. Although the researcher requests this clarification, it is heard by the co-present girls and provides for the girls the perspectives of their co-players. Reflecting on what occurs as part of accomplishing such requests for clarification highlights for me the requirement that the researcher is fully present with the children during the interview process and is following the unfolding interaction. Although at first this sounds unproblematic, in placing myself in the position of the researcher, I can see how there would be a number of considerations regarding, the planned schedule of questions, the video fragments and the unfolding talk. It highlights the delicate and intellectual work of supporting the co-construction of accounts with children, requiring careful planning and deep engagement in situ.

Third, the researcher draws on her 'professional stock of knowledge' (Peräkylä & Vehvil*f*inen, 2003) as a researcher and as a teacher, enabling child–child talk to unfold. In talk-in-interaction, the 'person who asks a question has a right to talk again' (Sacks, 1995: 49); however, in a multiparty setting, another person may self-select as a speaker. So, in account three, the researcher asks a clarification question and nominates the next speaker who takes a turn. Noticeable in this sequence is that the researcher does not interrupt the child–child interaction rather she lets the talk between the children escalate, and is an observer of the unfolding social order. As I read account three, I wondered how I might have responded given that a multiparty dispute unfolds and, as the researcher notes, it was a risky move. Although interested in how this is managed by the children, my sense is that the researcher would also have some concern about the wellbeing of the children, particularly given her previous role as an early childhood teacher where she would want to promote positive relationships. This move by the researcher leads to interesting insights into children's peer culture.

As a researcher of children's everyday lives in family and educational settings, as yet, I have not used video-stimulated accounts (Pomerantz, 2005; Theobald, 2012). This method enables children to provide their standpoint and have their views listened to (United Nations, 1989) and aligns well with my own commitment to childhood competence and participation, and I am now motivated to develop a research project that uses video-stimulated accounts.

Overall, this chapter highlights the problem facing researchers where they strive to give children a 'voice' in research and in particular, when tackling sensitive topics, such as disputes and breakdowns of friendships between peers. The voicing of children's standpoint is important as it provides children with an opportunity to share what is important to them. For researchers and people who work with young children, it provides a window into children's social world and the matters that impact them.

Researchers may encounter ethical dilemmas regarding wanting to learn more about sensitive issues to do with children's relationships, but need to minimize potential upsets to ensure children's wellbeing. There is much to learn about how to engage in this type of research from this chapter and the challenges faced by the researchers as they worked with the children.

Acknowledgements Thanks to the children and teacher involved in the study.

Funding A Research Capacity Building Scholarship from Queensland University of Technology (QUT) funded the original research, Children's participation in a preparatory classroom (Approval number 070000025). The Childhoods in Changing Contexts Research Group https://research.qut.edu.au/cccrg/ (QUT) supported the proofreading of the chapter.

Appendix 1: Transcription Notation

Gail Jefferson (2004) developed a transcription method to highlight the interactional features of conversational data. The following punctuation marks depict the characteristics of speech production, not the conventions of grammar, used in the transcripts.

did.	a full stop indicates a stopping fall in tone
here,	a comma indicates a continuing intonation
hey?	a question mark indicates a rising intonation
together!	an exclamation mark indicates an animated tone
you	underline indicates emphasis
¿	an inverted question mark indicates slightly rising intonation
°hey°	quiet speech
()	the talk is not audible
(house)	transcribers guess for the talk
⋮	a vertical ellipse indicates that intervening turns at talk have been omitted
(0.3)	number in second and tenths of a second indicates the length of an interval
So:::rry	colon represents a sound stretch
Dr-dirt	a single dash indicates a noticeable cut off of the prior word or sound
hhh	indicates an out-breath
.hhh	a dot prior to h indicates an in-breath
[hello]	brackets indicate overlapped speech
<stop>	speech is delivered slower than normal
>come<	speech is delivered faster than normal
funny	smiley voice
~upset~	tremulous voice

References

Antaki, C. (1994). *Explaining and arguing.* London: Sage.

Antaki, C. (2002). Personalized revision of 'failed' questions. *Discourse Studies, 4*(4), 411–428.

Bateman, A., & Danby, S. (2013). Recovering from the earthquake: Early childhood teachers and children collaboratively telling stories about their experiences. *Disaster Prevention and Management, 22*(5), 467–479.

Church, A. (2016). *Preference organisation and peer disputes: How young children resolve conflict.* London: Routledge.

Corsaro, W. A. (2017). *The sociology of childhood.* London: Sage.

Cromdal, J. (2004). Building bilingual oppositions: Code switching in children's disputes. *Language in Society, 33*(1), 33–58.

Daley, K. (2013). The wrongs of protection: Balancing protection and participation in research with marginalised young people. *Journal of Sociology*.
Danby, S. (2017). Technologies, child-centred practice and listening to children. In L. Arnott (Ed.), *Digital technology, play and learning in the early years* (pp. 127–139). London: Sage.
Danby, S., Ewing, L., & Thorpe, K. (2011). The novice researcher: Interviewing young children. *Qualitative Inquiry, 17*(1), 74–84.
Danby, S., & Farrell, A. (2005). Opening the research conversation. In A. Farrell (Ed.), *Ethical research with children* (pp. 49–67). Milton Keynes, Bucks: Open University Press.
Danby, S., & Theobald, M. (Eds.). (2012). *Disputes in everyday life: Social and moral orders of children and young people.* Sociological studies of children and youth (Special Volume 15). New York: Emerald.
Department of Education, Employment & Workforce Relations (DEEWR). (2009). *Belonging, being and becoming: The early years learning framework for Australia.* Canberra: Council of Australian Governments.
Dorner, L. M. (2014). From relating to (re)presenting: Challenges and lessons learned from an ethnographic study with young children. *Qualitative Inquiry, 21*(4), 345–365.
Early Childhood Australia (ECA). (2016). *Code of ethics.* Melbourne: Early Childhood Australia.
Edwards, D. (1999). Emotion discourse. *Culture & Psychology, 5*(3), 271–291.
Evaldsson, A. (2007). Accounting for friendship: Moral ordering and category membership in preadolescent girls' relational talk. *Research on Language and Social Interaction, 40*(4), 377–404.
Evang, A., & Øverlien, C. (2015). If you look, you have to leave?: Young children regulating research interviews about experiences of domestic violence. *Journal of Early Childhood Research, 13*(2), 113–125.
Farrell, A. (2016). Ethics in early childhood research. In A. Farrell, S. L. Kagan, & E. K. M. Tisdall (Eds.), *The SAGE handbook of early childhood research* (pp. 187–200). London: Sage.
Fitzgerald, R. (2012). Membership categorization analysis: Wild and promiscuous or simply the joy of Sacks? *Discourse Studies, 14*(3), 305–311.
Garfinkel, H. (1967). *Studies in ethnomethodology.* Englewood Cliffs, NJ: Prentice-Hall.
Gill, V. (1998). Doing attributions in medical interaction: Patients' explanations for illness and doctors' responses. *Social Psychology Quarterly, 61*(4), 342–360.
Goodwin, M. (1990). *He said—She said: Talk as social organization among black children.* Bloomington: Indiana University Press.

Goodwin, M., & Goodwin, C. (1987). Children's arguing. In S. U. Phillips, S. Steele, & C. Tanz (Eds.), *Language gender and sex in comparative perspectives* (pp. 200–248). Cambridge: Cambridge University Press.

Graham, A., & Fitzgerald, R. (2010). Progressing children's participation: Exploring the potential of a dialogical turn. *Childhood, 17*(3), 343–359.

Graham, A., Powell, M. A., & Taylor, N. (2015). Ethical research involving children: Encouraging reflexive engagement in research with children and young people. *Children and Society, 29*(5), 331–343.

Heritage, J. (1984). *Garfinkel and ethnomethodology*. Oxford: Polity Press.

Heritage, J. (1985). Analyzing news interviews: Aspects of the production of talk for an overhearing audience. In T. A. van Dijk (Ed.), *Handbook of discourse analysis, vol. 3: Discourse and dialogue* (pp. 95–117). London: Academic Press.

Heritage, J. (2002). The limits of questioning: Negative interrogatives and hostile question content. *Journal of Pragmatics, 34*(10–11), 1427–1446.

Heritage, J., & Watson, D. R. (1979). Formulations as conversational objects. In G. Psathas (Ed.), *Everyday language: Studies in ethnomethodology* (pp. 123–155). New York: Irvington Publishers.

Horgan, D. (2017). Child participatory research methods: Attempts to go 'deeper'. *Childhood, 24*(2), 245–259.

Hutchby, I. (2002). Resisting the incitement to talk in child counseling: Aspects of the utterance "I don't know". *Discourse Studies, 4*(2), 147–168.

Hutchby, I., & Moran-Ellis, J. (1998). Situating children's social competence. In I. Hutchby & J. Moran-Ellis (Eds.), *Children and social competence: Arenas of action* (pp. 7–26). London: Falmer Press.

Jefferson, G. (2004). Glossary of transcript symbols with an Introduction. In G. Lerner (Ed.), *Conversation analysis: Studies from the first generation* (pp. 13–23). Philadelphia: John Benjamins.

Lamerichs, J., Alisic, E., & Schasfoort, M. (2018). Accounts and their epistemic implications: How children's '*I don't know*' answers are received in trauma recovery talk. *Research on Children and Social Interaction, 2*(1), 25–48.

Mackay, R. (1991). Conceptions of children and models of socialisation. In F. C. Waksler (Ed.), *Studying the social worlds of children: Sociological readings* (pp. 23–37). London: Falmer Press.

Mason, J., & Danby, S. (2011). Editorial to special issue: Children as experts in their lives: Child inclusive research. *Child Indicators Research, 4*(2), 185–189.

Maynard, D. W. (1985a). How children start arguments. *Language in Society, 14*(1), 1–30.

Maynard, D. W. (1985b). On the functions of social conflict among children. *American Sociological Review, 50*(2), 207–223.

Maynard, D. W. (1986). Offering and soliciting collaboration in multi-party disputes among children (and other humans). *Human Studies, 9*(2–3), 261–285.
Mayne, F., Howitt, C., & Rennie, L. J. (2018). A hierarchical model of children's research participation rights based on information, understanding, voice, and influence. *European Early Childhood Education Research Journal, 26*(5), 644–656.
O'Reilly, M., Lester, J. N., & Muskett, T. (2016). Children's claims to knowledge regarding their mental health experiences and practitioner's negotiation of the problem. *Patient Education and Counseling, 99*(6), 905–910.
Peräkylä, A., & Vehvilƒinen, S. (2003). Conversation analysis and the professional stocks of interactional knowledge. *Discourse & Society, 14*(6), 727–750.
Pomerantz, A. (2005). Using participants' video stimulated comments to complement analyses of interactional practices. In H. te Molder & J. Potter (Eds.), *Conversation and cognition* (pp. 93–113). Cambridge: Cambridge University Press.
Powell, S., & Anderson, C. (2005). Ethical aspects of power in research with children. In A. Farrell (Ed.), *Ethical research with children* (pp. 124–138). London: McGraw-Hill.
Prout, A., & James, A. (1997). A new paradigm for the sociology of childhood? Provenance, promise and problems. In A. James & A. Prout (Eds.), *Constructing and reconstructing childhood: Contemporary issues in the sociological study of childhood* (pp. 7–34). London: Falmer Press.
Psathas, G. (1992). The study of extended sequences: The case of the garden lesson. In G. Watson & R. Seiler (Eds.), *Text in context: Contributions to ethnomethodology* (pp. 99–122). Newbury Park: Sage.
Quennerstedt, A., & Quennerstedt, M. (2014). Researching children's rights in education: Sociology of childhood encountering educational theory. *British Journal of Sociology of Education, 35*(1), 115–132.
Sacks, H. (1972). On the analyzability of stories by children. In J. J. Gumperz & D. Hymes (Eds.), *Directions in sociolinguistic: The ethnography of communication* (pp. 325–345). Cambridge: Cambridge University Press.
Sacks, H. (1995). *Lectures on conversation (Vols. I & II).* Malden, MA: Blackwell.
Sharpe, V. A. (1997). Why "do no harm"? *Theoretical Medicine, 18*(1–2), 197–215.
Sidnell, J., & Stivers, T. (Eds.). (2012). *The handbook of conversation analysis.* Malden: Blackwell.
Silverman, D. (1987). *Communication and medical practice: Social relations in the clinic.* London: Sage.

Skelton, T. (2008). Research with children and young people: Exploring the tensions between ethics, competence and participation. *Children's Geographies, 6*(1), 21–36.

Speier, M. (1973). *How to observe face-to-face communication: A sociological introduction.* Pacific Palisades, CA: Goodyear Publishing.

Theobald, M. (2012). Video-stimulated accounts: Young children accounting for interactional matters in front of peers. *Journal of Early Childhood Research, 10*(1), 32–50.

Theobald, M. (2017). Children as research participants in educational research using video-stimulated accounts. *International Journal of Educational Research, 86,* 131–143.

Theobald, M., & Danby, S. (2017). Co-producing cultural knowledge: Children telling tales in the school playground. In A. Bateman & A. Church (Eds.), *Children's knowledge-in-interaction: Studies in conversation analysis* (pp. 111–125). Singapore: Springer.

Theobald, M., Danby, S., & Ailwood, J. (2011). Child participation in the early years: Challenges for education. *Australasian Journal of Early Childhood, 36*(3), 19–26.

Tisdall, E. M. (2016). Participation, rights and 'participatory' methods. In A. Farrell, S. L. Kagan, & E. K. M. Tisdall (Eds.), *The SAGE handbook of early childhood research* (pp. 73–88). London: Sage.

United Nations. (1989). *Convention on the rights of the child.* Retrieved 26 June 2015, from http://www.ohchr.org/english/law/crc.htm.

7

'Well I Had Nothing Weird Going On': Children's Displays of Social Competence in Psychological Research Interviews

Joyce Lamerichs, Eva Alisic and Marca Schasfoort

Professional Reflection by Eva Alisic

Introduction

Conversation analytic studies of professional-child interactions have shown that children are able to employ their knowledge of a particular institutional environment to manage their interactional space. Children may create and maintain this interactional space in diverse settings and participation frameworks, and by instantiating a range of conversational practices. Practices of resistance have been well-documented, for example,

J. Lamerichs (✉) · M. Schasfoort
Department of Language, Literature and Communication, VU University Amsterdam, Amsterdam, The Netherlands
e-mail: j.m.w.j.lamerichs@vu.nl

M. Schasfoort
e-mail: m.c.g.schasfoort@vu.nl

J. Lamerichs et al. (eds.), *Children and Mental Health Talk*, The Language of Mental Health,
https://doi.org/10.1007/978-3-030-28426-8_7

in educational and counselling settings (Danby & Baker, 1998; Hutchby, 2005, 2007), as well as practices in which resistance strategies go hand in hand with aligning with the professional or even accommodating to what the interviewer wants to hear. This is shown to be the case in judicial interviews and interviews that discuss sensitive topics such as sexual abuse or domestic violence (Childs & Walsh, 2017; Iversen, 2014; van Nijnatten, 2013).

This chapter starts from the idea that children employ conversational practices like the above to constitute their social competence in interaction with professionals. We propose that children do so as members of the 'indigenous language cultures of childhood, which can be more or less independent of adults' (Hutchby, 2005: 71). We also put a relational and conversational concept of children's competence centre stage, rather than a cognitively or individually based, more static definition (Clark & Richards, 2017).

Children's interactional displays of competence are explored when they are invited to participate in a psychological research interview with a trained psychologist. These research interviews have been undertaken as part of a larger study to find out how children have experienced recuperation from instances of 'single-incident trauma', and with the explicit aim to advance a more child-oriented perspective on trauma recovery (Alisic, Boeije, Jongmans, & Kleber, 2011; Van Wesel, Boeije, Alisic, & Drost, 2012). To acquire the perspective of the child was considered especially important because the field of trauma-informed care is still largely dominated by studies that focus on adults who may experience and process traumatic events differently when compared to children.

For this chapter, we have analysed interviews that concern the sudden loss of a parent or sibling through an accident, experiences of violence in the family (murder), and experiences of personal violence (sexual assault) that satisfied the A1 exposure criterion for Posttraumatic Stress Disorder in

---

E. Alisic
Melbourne School of Population and Global Health, University of Melbourne, Melbourne, VIC, Australia
e-mail: ealisic@unimelb.edu.au

the Diagnostic and Statistical Manual of Mental Disorders (APA, 2000). At the time of the interviews, the children were no longer receiving mental health care. During the interviews, a semi-structured approach was used in which the children were invited to describe their view of what happened, its aftermath and how they have experienced the process of recovery.

Although the interviews cover a broad set of traumatic occurrences, the aim of this chapter is to determine whether there are routine ways in which children are invited to talk about these experiences in this interview setting. In particular, our analysis focuses on how children manage the interactional implications of this setting in which situationally relevant notions such as 'change' and 'recovery' are introduced by the professional, as they constitute relevant categories for the original interview study (Alisic et al., 2011). Our aim is to investigate how given such institutional goals, children respond to the above notions that are embedded in the question format. The data offer a valuable opportunity to further develop our knowledge of research interviews in what can be considered a sensitive context (see also Lamerichs, Alisic, & Schasfoort, 2018) as well as to detail some of the challenges of qualitative methods such as interviewing as a means to gather insights in children's experiences or perspectives (Blakely & Moles, 2016; Silverman, 2017).

Our analyses are guided by a conversation analytic (hence CA) perspective and by insights from discursive psychology (hence DP), most notably the work on how speakers handle issues of accountability and morality in talk (Bergmann, 1998; Buttny, 2003). In line with these interactional approaches, we consider interviews based on information seeking questions not as 'pathways' to children's thoughts and feelings, but as sites for action, identity work and co-construction in the light of their institutionally relevant goals (Freed & Ehrlich, 2010; Potter & Hepburn, 2005; also Iversen, 2014: 368; see also Lamerichs, Alisic, & Schasfoort, 2015).

Theoretical Section

Institutional settings in which children and professionals take part, such as child counselling or family therapy, can be characterised by differing interactional agendas and differing moral imperatives. The notion of moral imperatives can be drawn on in at least two ways. In a first and general sense, it may be related to institutionally specific question formats and how such formats reflect 'institutional moral frameworks' (Freed & Ehrlich, 2010). Such moral frameworks seem to be bound up with an organisation's institutional remit. In divorce counselling with children, for example, the notion of moral frameworks relates to the conversational practices used by the professional to engage in counselling-relevant tasks (Hutchby, 2005). Children may not always comply with such tasks, interactionally. For example, it was shown how the moral framework that was implied by the counsellor's questions (such as inviting the child to engage in 'feelings talk') was resisted by the child.

Questions asked in family therapy sessions, where generally both the parents and the child are present, offer another illustration of how institutional moral frameworks constitute an interactional concern for participants. Questions asked by the therapist in these settings might carry specific moral reflections, such as being a 'bad' child or a 'good' parent. When the therapist seeks a particular account about whether the child feels victimised by his parents, the parents may offer an account of 'good parenthood' in response instead. Producing such an account allows parents to counter the specific negative moral reflections in the question, whereas the space for the child to respond is limited (Hutchby, 2015; Hutchby & O'Reilly, 2010: 55–56; see also Bergmann, 1998, for a full discussion on accounts).

Our analysis of the data from psychological research interviews aims to explore how children attend to questions asked by the interviewer, that are couched in terms of institutionally relevant notions such as 'change' or 'recovery'. We want to explore how children manage the possible moral reflections in these (prefaced) questions (section "Presenting Downgraded Versions of What Happened") and the identity work they engage in while doing so. We also aim to expand our knowledge of what it means when we invite children to speak about traumatic experience from the perspective of change and recovery via psychological interviews (cf. Potter & Hepburn, 2005), while our analysis will also highlight some of the moral categories children themselves draw on in their answers (section "Discounting Ascriptions of a Changed Self"). We first discuss the characteristics of question formats and their institutional specificities.

The Institutional Specificity of Question Design

The premises of question design in professional-child interaction are well worth exploring in our data (see also Lamerichs et al., 2015, 2018) and have been extensively examined in CA (Freed & Ehrlich, 2010; also Heritage, 2010). Studies have demonstrated how question design is related to the professional roles of the interactants (e.g. as a doctor, counsellor, or in our case, a trained psychologist), and how this shows up in the structure, lexical formatting and presuppositional basis of questions (Boyd & Heritage, 2006). Analyses of doctor-patient interaction provide an apt illustration here, as the questions doctors pose may be formatted in structurally different terms than the patient's responses. Where doctors may ask a question that searches for quantifiable measures of certain behaviour (e.g. alcohol consumption in terms of *units per week*), patients may answer such a question by offering qualitative biographical detail (i.e. describing alcohol consumption as part of their lifestyle, irrespective of numbers, see Halkowski, 1998). Thus, where doctors (and psychologists) might be trained to use objective measures in the formatting of their questions to arrive at appropriate assessments of relevant lifestyle factors, patients, on the other hand, may describe such factors in a context of sociability. Providing such biographical detail is interactionally relevant, as it wards off a 'technical' description of alcohol use that may suggest an overt monitoring of alcohol intake (see also Halkowski, 2006 on how patients' descriptions strike a balance between paying too much and too little attention to their bodily condition).

We see similar instances of institutionally relevant question design in our data, most notably with respect to the interviewer's questions inquiring about aspects of 'change', as a result of the traumatic occurrence (see also Urman, Funk, & Elliot, 2001 for questions typically asked in interviews to elicit children's stories on traumatic experiences). Previous work has shown how the questions in these interviews have a complex, often prefaced design (Lamerichs et al., 2018). Our data show that these prefaced question formats may be used to introduce a hypothetical scenario (e.g. 'sometimes children experience something bad like that and then afterwards they view the world in a different light how is that for you', see Fragments 2 and 3). These hypothetical scenarios make answer positions available that are tilted in favour of a confirming response because a possible change in world view is made relevant and recognisable as something that happens to children in a similar situation. Other fragments also make available presuppositions and invite to confirm, for example, when inquiring about 'a changed view of the world' ('don't you view the world differently', in Fragments 4 and 5).

We inspect the interactional consequences of such question formats and how in answering these questions, children manage to talk about their traumatic experiences *in their own words*, and what these words demonstrably counter or resist.

Managing 'Normality' and 'Difference'

Not much is known about the ways in which children talk about their experiences with traumatic events. However, a content analysis of therapeutic trauma interviews with children shows that children strongly orient to categories of 'normality' and 'difference' as two broad frames of reference to make sense of their experiences during and after a traumatic experience (Urman et al., 2001); a finding that is also consistent with earlier research (Terr, 1990). Conversation analytic studies have also found 'normalising' strategies at work, which have been termed 'doing being ordinary' (Sacks, 1984). These strategies are attended to in different settings and in different ways. When interviewed about alleged sexual abuse by a social worker, children may describe their experiences as quite 'ordinary' or 'temporary', and not in need of particular professional attention (van Nijnatten, 2013). When asked to report on their experiences of alleged sexual abuse by a police officer, victims also produce descriptions that 'normalise' the event, or render it a 'non-problem event' (Kidwell, 2009: 28). A similar concern with 'doing being ordinary' has been demonstrated in settings in which participants find themselves in a situation of 'social evaluation'. When interviewed by a social worker about adoptive parenthood, couples may describe themselves as 'normal' people who have had 'normal' childhoods (Noordegraaf, Van Nijnatten, & Elbers, 2009).

How 'normality', and by implication 'abnormality', work as performative categories has also been addressed in paediatric therapy interactions that involve children with autism (Lester, 2014). In interactions with caretakers, professionals typically engage in practices that explain the behaviour of the child as meaningful and relevant, thereby redefining which behaviour might fall outside 'the norm' and for whom. Hence, attributions of competence and normality are shaped in interactions, illustrating again how a particular institutional moral framework is talked into being in this setting (2014: 179).

We argue that the interviewer questions that inquire about 'change' or 'recovery' in our interview data are equally not neutral or objective requests for information, but make available particular institutionally relevant answer agendas and are imbued with moral implications (Hutchby, 2005; Hutchby and O'Reilly, 2010). We will demonstrate how children may resist some of these moral implications (e.g. by downplaying the suggestion of fundamental change as a result of what happened), while they may also be shown to do moral work themselves (e.g. by emphasising their success in—having learned—to live a 'normal life' again). Examining these interactional practices enables us to detail children's differential displays of social competence in the setting of the psychological research interview.

Data, Method and Approach

Our analysis draws on semi-structured psychological research interviews that were conducted for a qualitative study on child trauma. The aim of the original study was to examine how children experience the recovery process after a traumatic event and which factors they themselves identify as helping or hindering. Twenty-five children (15 boys and 10 girls, aged 8–12 years) participated in the study, who experienced different types of trauma, classified elsewhere as falling under the categories of sudden loss, violence and accidents with injury (see Alisic et al., 2011 for a full account of the study). The events had occurred between ten months and seven years previously, with a median of 27 months.

The children and their parents had been recruited via records held by the University Medical Center Utrecht in the Netherlands, with approval of its medical ethics committee for the study protocol. Children who had been confronted with a single-incident trauma were eligible for the study if they were aged between eight and twelve, if they were not currently receiving mental health care, and if the event had occurred at least six months previously. The research team recruited families by letter and called them to answer any questions. Written informed consent and verbal assent were obtained from the parents and the children, respectively. The study made use of purposive sampling to achieve a maximum range in demographic characteristics, types of trauma, time since trauma, and degree of mental health care. For the current analysis, we examine the interviews of the 13 children whose families approved secondary use of the interviews for research purposes.

The interviews with the children were all conducted by the same interviewer (and co-author of this chapter, EA), who is a trained psychologist, in a quiet room and separate from their parents. Most of the interviews took place in one of the playrooms in the Medical Center, while a few were conducted, at the family's request, in their home. Several measures were taken to make the child feel at ease and in control, such as play at the beginning of the interview and a stop sign (a copy of the traffic sign) that the child could use to terminate the interview. None of the children used the sign or other means to terminate the interview prematurely. The interviews included the following topics: the characteristics of the trauma, the child's immediate reactions, how the child's reactions evolved over time, to what extent the child experienced changes in outlook on the world, the self or others, what self-identified milestones had occurred in the child's recovery, and factors that had assisted or impeded recovery.

The purpose of the interviews was to learn about the child's view and to limit the amount of influence on the child's responses while eliciting as much information as possible. The research team continuously adapted the interview questions based on themes that emerged during the study. The body of the interviews (excluding play, introduction, and ending) lasted 30 minutes on average.

This study employs an interactional approach, building on insights in CA and DP that are used to explore interactional practices in medical settings as well as other institutional environments that involve children (O'Reilly & Lester, 2015; also Hutchby & Woofitt, 2008). Based on fine-grained analyses, these interactional approaches allow for a systematic exploration of how speakers display their understandings of what they are saying and doing, as evidenced in the local particularities of talk. Detailed transcripts of the talk at hand are used, based on guidelines conventionally adopted in CA (Jefferson, 2004).

For this chapter, we report on the findings from a selection of 6 interviews that are concerned with experiences of violence and loss. Based on this dataset, our collection study was informed by three broad sets of identified practices that children seemed to engage in and which may fall under the larger interactional project of 'doing being ordinary'. In the analysis that follows, we present the original data in Dutch and a gloss in English.[1]

Analysis

Our analysis focuses on how children engage in answering a particular set of questions that highlight institutionally relevant notions of personal change or a changed outlook on life. Section "Presenting Downgraded Versions of What Happened" presents how in response to such questions, children construct what happened to them in a downgraded fashion or resist the implication of personal change.

Section "Discounting Ascriptions of a Changed Self" highlights how children, in response to questions that inquire about 'changes' as a result of what has happened, emphasise their 'regained normality'. In doing so, they actively resist the implication that what happened to them has caused them to change as a person. Lastly, section "Presenting Normatively Preferred Versions of 'Doing Being Recovered'" examines how children themselves also engage in 'moral work', when presenting normatively preferred accounts of 'doing being recovered'. Together these practices show how children engage in identity work, vis-à-vis the questions that are posed to them in this setting, which inquire to recount past experiences in the here and now.

[1] We provide a two-line transcript including the Dutch originals and an idiomatic English translation that attempts to capture the local interactional meaning of the original utterance in Dutch. We convey the English translations without production details within lexical items as we cannot 'translate' how these features would be rendered by the speakers in English (Hepburn & Bolden, 2013). Pauses, speed, volume, turn-initial in breath and indicators of turn-final intonation are however included in the translations. With turn-final intonation, we follow the guidelines by Mazeland (2003), who uses the semicolon to identify a pitch rise stronger than a comma but weaker than a question mark (cf. 2013: 61–62).

Presenting Downgraded Versions of What Happened

Fragment 1 occurs in the first minutes of an interview with a girl who was abducted and sexually assaulted by an unknown man. The interviewer has just started off the interview by asking the child to tell 'the story of what happened' (data not shown here). At the start of Fragment 1, the girl told the interviewer how she was eventually taken back to the community centre by someone from her village who saw her sitting in a nearby park while her family was looking for her.

Fragment 1

```
k22 - 'well I had nothing weird going on'
80 I:  en weet je nog (.)
       and do you still know (.)
81 I:  hoe het toen met jou was.
       how it was then with you.
82 I:  °toen je terug ging naar de club°.=
       °when you went back to the community centre°=
83 K:  =NOU (.) i:k (.) h wist niet echt wat er gebeurde;
       =WELL (.) I (.) did not really know what was happening;
84 K:  [want ik was zes.
       [because I was six years old.
85 I:  [°nee°;
       [°no°;
86     [((bladeren-ritselen van papier))]
       [((leafing through - rustling of sheets of paper))]
87 I:  ja:;
       yes:;
88 K:  dan snap je dat ook niet e↑cht,
       then you don't really understand those things,
89 I:  mhnee.
       mhno.
90     (2.0)
91 I:  weet je nog hoe je je toen ↑voe:lde,
       do you still know how you felt at the time,
92     (0.5)
93 K:  hh↑m.
       hhm.
94     (0.5)
95 K:  nou ik had niks rAA:↑rs;
       well I had nothing wEIrd going on;
96 K:  want    [.hh (1.0)
       because [.hh (1.0)
97 I:          [hh↑m
               [hhm
98 K:  ik wist niet ee(h)ns w(h)at er- dat er iets aan de hand was.
       I did not even know what was- that something was going on.
99 I:  nee;
       no;
```

In lines 80–82, the interviewer formulates a polar question ('do you still know how..'), that inquires how the child 'was' at that moment ('how it was then with you…', line 81) when she was taken back to the community centre. The presuppositional basis of the question is that something about the child's situation at that moment is relevant to report on here. And also, that it is relevant not so much to report on it in neutral terms but as a possible 'problem event' (Kidwell, 2009: 23). The child's answer starts with the discourse marker 'well', which is attended to in a way that is in line with Schegloff and Lerner's observations (2009) on the use of well-prefacing in response to wh-questions: it is not produced as a dispreference marker but as an alert that something is the matter with how the speaker is continuing the turn (cf. Mazeland, 2016). She continues by producing an epistemic disclaimer that wards off being actively aware of the nature of what happened, which she then accounts for (in overlap with a confirmation from the interviewer) in terms of her young age (line 84). This account, which makes use of a stage-of-life categorisation, is followed by an elaboration that upgrades the categorisation into a more generic claim: no one can be expected to understand the act of being sexually assaulted at such an early age (see the use of 'you', in line 88; see Cromdal, Danby, Emmison, Osvaldsson, & Cobb-Moore, 2017).

After a confirming response, the interviewer continues in line 91 by inquiring how the child *felt* at the time (note the polar design, similar to lines 80–81, starting with '*do you still know*'). The child responds again with the discourse marker 'well', which highlights that what comes next is not straightforward (Mazeland, 2016): she goes on to reject the possible inference that something was observably 'wrong' with her then ('well I had nothing weird going on', line 52, said in a louder voice and with emphasis). This is then coupled with an account that contains an 'extremised' epistemic disclaimer ('I did not even know', in line 98), produced with laughter particles. Thus, the child counters the suggestion of being aware of what exactly happened when she was abducted, nor of any possible ramifications, which downplays its importance and renders it a *non*-problematic event. The trajectory of the interviewer's questions, presupposing at two instances that the child's mental state at the time is relevant to report on here, is resisted. Note that the girl's accounts in lines 83 and 98, which all work to counter the presuppositional basis of the question, can also be heard as subtly criticising the basis for the interviewer's question.

Fragment 2 below presents an fragment from an interview with another girl who was raped by a young boy from her hometown. The interviewer poses a lengthy prefaced question, which is not displayed in full here. It outlines a scenario in which other children who have also experienced 'something really bad', still have a feeling that there is something positive about what has happened to them (lines 726–728). Its format presumes the likelihood of a similar experience and seeks confirmation from the girl. After a 2.6 second break, in which the girl has not responded, the interviewer asks the child 'how' that has been for her (line 730, see also Fragment 3 for a similar question design).

Fragment 2

```
k20 - 'it could also have happened to someone else'
726 I: .hh en dan hebben ze t↑och nog het gev↑oel,
       .hh and then they still have the feeling,
727 I: .h dat er ↑iets posit↓iefs;
       .h that there has been something positive;
728 I: is geweest °aan de gebeurtenis°.
       °about the occurrence°.
729    (2.6)
730 I: °hoe was dat bij jou°.
       °how was that with you°.
731 K: °hm°
       °hm°
732    (3.0)
733 K: ja;
       yes;
734    (1.0)
735 K: weet ik niet echt.
       I don't really know.
736 K: [ja;]
       [yes;]
737 I: [nee] 't hoeft niet he;
       [no] it doesn't have to be does it;
738    (1.8)
739 K: nee volgens mij heb ik dat niet echt.
       no I don't think I really have that.
740 I: nee;
       no;
741 K: het is wel vervelend=
       it is unpleasant=
742 K: =maar,
       =but,
743 I: hmhm;
       hmhm;
744 K: het had ook bij iemand anders kunnen gebeuren.
       it could also have happened to someone else.
```

```
745 I: ja;
       yes;
746    (2.5)
747 I: wat bedoel je daar precies mee?
       what exactly do you mean by that?
748 K: nou;
       well;
749    (2.0)
750 K: pt a- eh eh die jongen had ook gewoon iemand
       pt a- uh uh that boy could also have just
751 K: a↑nders kunnen roepen;
       called on someone else;
752 I: [hmhm]
       [hmhm]
753 K: [en had] dan ook gewoon iemand a↑nders >kunnen verkrachten<.
       [and could] then also just have raped someone else.
754 I: ja.=
       yes.=
755 K: =dus (.) o- misschien was het dan wel met m-m'n vriendin gebeurd.
       =so (.) o- maybe it would have happened to my girlfriend then.
756 I: hmhm;
       hmhm;
757    (3.0)
758 K: °dus°(1.0) soms zijn dingen ook gewoon zo;
       °so° (1.0) sometimes things are also just like that;
759 K: zoals het is.
       the way it is.
760 I: ja.
       yes.
761    (4.0)
```

In response to the interviewer's 'how' question in line 730, the child responds with markers of hesitance and an epistemic disclaimer ('don't really know', line 735; see also Lamerichs et al., 2018; also Stafford, Hutchby, Karim, & O'Reilly, 2016). The interviewer produces a confirmation in overlap with the child and an acknowledgement that this does not necessarily have to be the case and seeks confirmation from the child (line 737). The child confirms this acknowledgement by stating more explicitly that she has not taken something positive from what happened. She continues by producing two further statements that describe the nature of the occurrence in a downgraded fashion ('it is unpleasant'; 'it could also have happened to someone else', lines 741–744). These downgraded descriptions may be hearable as a disagreeing with the question that what happened to her falls under the 'special' category of events that, in retrospect, would allow for anything positive to be gained from it. After a confirmation, the interviewer asks a follow-up question for clarification (line 747). In response, the child offers a well-prefaced answer that uses a hypothetical construction with multiple references to the adverb 'just' to highlight the coincidental nature of what happened. The use of the turn-initial 'well' ('nou' in Dutch) in this question-answer sequence is another example (see also Fragment 2) of how some uses of 'well' may not be particularly governed by participant orientations to a preferred or dispreferred response (Mazeland, 2016). It seems to be oriented to how her 'response will be in some respect not straightforward' (Schegloff & Lerner, 2009: 101).

By formulating that 'sometimes things are also just like that' (line 758) she then does closing work to present what happened to her in a matter-of-fact fashion. It is presented as an occurrence she is now able to reflect on and as a fact of life that lies in the past, rather than it being in need of any further contemplation in the here and now. In doing so, the child's answer may subtly resist the trajectory of the question that inquires how this particular experience may be of the life-changing kind from which one is able to distil particular positive lessons.

In this section, we have examined two fragments in which two girls who experienced rape and sexual assault respectively, are invited to tell the story of what happened. Both fragments have shown how the girls subtly resist the trajectory of the question that inquires into whether there was something observably 'strange' (or 'wrong') after what happened; the traumatic event is presented in downgraded and ordinary terms. Fragment 2 also demonstrated that what happened is attended to as something that does not warrant any further contemplation, and so continued topicalisation of this matter in the terms the question poses, is resisted. Next we will examine how the children in our data actively counter the suggestion of a 'changed self', as a result of what happened. We gloss this as another way in which children instantiate 'doing being ordinary'.

Discounting Ascriptions of a Changed Self

The fragments in this section deal with the topical agenda of one of the interviewer's questions that inquires about 'changes' that have occurred since the traumatic event. These questions were sometimes asked on multiple occasions during the interview. Fragment 3 explores how this question gets responded to by the girl who was sexually assaulted (Fragment

1), and we continue by showing how other children may also resist the topical agenda of changes to the self, as a result of what happened.

Fragment 3 below shows a similar question format we saw at the start of Fragment 2. The interviewer starts with a prefaced question design that invites confirmation, as it stresses the likelihood that a changed world view is in order. In line 330, the preface is coupled with a 'how' question, which, based on the assumptions in the preface, may make a confirmation from the child relevant.

Fragment 3

k22 - 'I am still just the same person'

```
324 I:  .hh hee en soms dan eh maken kinderen zoiets ergs ↑mee,
        .hh hey and sometimes children experience something bad like that,
325 K:  hmhm.
        hmhm.
326 I:  •pt en dan kijken ze daarna op een andere manier naar de ↓wereld;
        •pt and then afterwards they view the world in a different light;
327 I:  en naar mensen om hun heen;
        and the people around them;
328     (.)
329 I:  .h
        .h
330 I:  hoe is dat voor jou;
        how is that for you;
331     (1.0)
332 K:  nou:;
        well;
333 K:  ik let nu wel iets meer o:p,
        I do pay a little more attention now,
334 K:  maar; .h=
        but; .h=
335 I:  =huhhmm,
        =huhhmm,
336 K:  i:k kijk niet anders >naar de wereld ofzo<.
        I don't view the world differently or something.
337 I:  nee.
        no.
338 I:  °↑oke.°
        °okay°
339 K:  ik ben nog steeds gewoo:n
        I am still just
340     (0.5)
341 K:  hetze(h)lfde perso(h)on.
        the same person.
342 I:  ↑hmhm:m,
        ↑hmhm:m,
```

In lines 332–333 and after a one-second pause, the child responds with what begins with a weak agreement (Pomerantz, 1984) that points to a small change in behaviour. Note how the well-prefaced response might indicate that the answer that is forthcoming is not straightforward (Mazeland, 2016). The turn gets constructed as a contrast, in which the first part is presented as slightly different current behaviour of the child, without explicitly linking it to what happened. After a confirming response by the interviewer, the girl then continues with the but-prefaced second part of her answer that disconfirms that a more fundamental type of change is in order (line 336). After the interviewer's continuer and an 'okay' which might be hearable as another continuer or as doing closing work, the child goes on to emphasise her 'sameness' in stronger ('still') and normalising ('just') terms (in lines 339–341). This is then met with another continuer from the interviewer.

Similar practices to discount the question's topical agenda that inquires after personal change can be found in other interviews too. In Fragments 4 and 5 below, we present further examples from two interviews with two young boys. The boy in Fragment 4 has lost his father to suicide and the boy in Fragment 5 has lost his sister as a result of a train accident.

Prior to the beginning of Fragment 4, the interviewer has asked the boy whether things have changed following his father's death. The boy responds that their home had been redecorated and there is some laughter when he offers some evaluative remarks about this change ('to be honest it is prettier', data not shown here). The fragment starts when the interviewer asks a follow-up question that explicitly inquires whether the redecorating was directly related to his father's death (lines 519–520). After the boy produces a disconfirming response, in overlap and with laughter in line 521, the interviewer continues with what is presented as the second part to the alternative question ('or is that just unrelated', line 522). Formatted as more congruent with the boy's intervening response in line 521, and formatted as a more 'plausible' answer category ('just', line 522), it invites a confirmation from the boy.

Fragment 4

```
k8 - 'actually not so much had changed'
519  I:   en had dat ook te ma↑:ken met je vade↑r,
          and was that also related to your dad,
520  I:   dat dat nu [veranderd is
          that that has now [changed
521  K:              [ehh nee (h)h.
                          [ehh no (h)h.
522  I:   of is dat gewoo:n: los [van elkaar.]
          or  is  that  just not [connected to it.] (.)
523  K:                          [ehm nee ehh] (.)
                                 [ehm nee ehh] (.)
524  K:   .h hh >nee er was eigenlijk< niet zovee:l °veranderd°.
          .h hh >actually< not so much had changed.
525  I:   hmhm
          hmhm
526       (.)
527  I:   °oke°
          °okay°
528  I:   .h en: zijn er nog dinge' voor jou veranderd;
          .h and are there things for you that have changed;
529  I:   in hoe je (.) over andere dinge' denkt?
          in how you think about other things?
530       (3.0)
531  K:   nee: ook nie' °nee°.
          no not either no.
532  I:   nee, (.)[kijk je niet anders] naar de we:reld
          no, (.) [don't you look differently upon the world
533  I:   of naar mense:'.
          or people.
534  K:   [°niet echt nee°.
          [°not really no°.
535  K:   nee.
          no.
536  I:   °oke°
          °okay°
537       (2.5)
538  I:   °da' kan soms°;
          °that is possible sometimes°;
```

In lines 521 and 523, the boy replies with an overlapping and disconfirming 'no' and elaborates by downplaying the extent of the redecoration of his home. By adding the adverb 'actually' the boy's response counters the presuppositional basis of the question, that there had been made changes in the home, where a confirmation might be invited (Clift, 2001). After the interviewer's 'okay', which does closing work and paves the way for an and-prefaced follow-up question (Beach, 1993), the interviewer now renders the question more specific. She inquires whether any changes have occurred that have to do with the boy himself and how he thinks about 'other things' (lines 528–529). The boy produces a disconfirming 'no' that orients to these other dimensions of change that are asked about (line

531 'no not either no') which is repeated. The interviewer then rephrases the question in line 532, as a negative interrogative (Heritage, 2002), which invites a confirming response. The boy, again, produces a slightly weaker but still disconfirming response that gets softer produced (line 534) and repeated. In lines 536, the interviewer then offers an 'okay' in third position, which is also softer produced with which she seems to mildly acknowledge the plausibility of the boy's answer ('that is possible sometimes').

In Fragment 5, we present another example of a question that inquires about change as result of what happened. The interview is ten minutes under way, in which the interviewer asks about the changes since the boy's sister passed away as the result of an accident. In lines 582–583, the interviewer starts with a question design that highlights the self as the area where changes are sought ('are there things that have changed with you', line 582, see also Fragment 4, line 526). Similar to the previous fragments we have seen, the question makes available the topical agenda of 'personal change', as a result of the traumatic occurrence.

Fragment 5

```
k10 - 'so that has actually remained the same'
582  I:  zijn er dingen bij jou veranderd,
         are there things that have changed with you,
583  I:  in hoe je (0.8) na:denkt over- (0,8) dingen in de wereld?
         in how you (0.8) think about the things in the world?
584      (1.3)
585  K:  °nee°
         °no°
586  K:  [((smakt))] gewoon;
         [((smacks lips))] just;
587  K:  >altijd wachten bij het stoplicht,
         >always wait at the traffic lights,
588  K:  en bij het spoor<,
         and at the tracks<,
589  K:  ((dat)) doe ik ook altijd;
         I always do that too;
590  I:  hm mm
         hm mm
591  K:  .h en dee ik daarv↑oor ook al.
         .h and I used to do that too.
592  I:  okee.
         okay.
593      (0.4)
594  I:  dus dat is eigenlijk utzelfde gebleven,
         so that has actually remained the same,
595      (0.4))
596  K:  jha.
         yeah.
597      (1.4)
```

598 I: en zijn er dingen ook nog wel veranderd?
and are there also things that have changed?
599 (1.6)
600 K: eehm;
eehm;
601 (2.5)
602 K: n:ee.
no.
603 (2.3)
604 K: nou::,(°<dat we>°) wel verdrietig zijn.
well::,(°that we°>) are sad after all.
605 I: jha.
yeah.
606 (4.6)
607 I: °maar wat is daaraan veranderd;°
°but what has changed about that;°
608 (2.7)
609 K: nou ((dat)) wee ik nie.
well (that) I don't know.
610 I: hm mm
hm mm
611 (2.1)
612 I: °.hokee;°
°.hokay;°
613 (0.8)

After a pause and some markers of hesitance, the boy responds in lines 585–588 with a disconfirming answer followed by a 'just'-prefaced elaboration that presents 'ordinary behaviour' (i.e. waiting for the traffic lights and at the tracks). He then goes on to reformulate his answer by presenting this behaviour as something he always does (line 589) and then further retracts it by stating that this is also what he did before the accident (line 591), thus establishing it, in retrospect, as *un*changed behaviour, which is confirmed by the interviewer's formulation in line 594. The interviewer initiates a follow-up question that inquires whether there were things that '*have* change' (note the emphasis in Dutch, line 598). We see again some markers of hesitation, the start of a disconfirming response ('no') which then after a gap continuous with a stretched turn-initial 'well' which can be heard, not so much as a dispreference marker, but indicating a complicated answer. It is produced in unforeseen terms to indicate change in the sense that the family has been sad (line 604). Without an acknowledgement, but with a softer produced 'but'-prefaced follow-up question, the interviewer seems to treat this answer as not completely sufficient and asks for a respecification of the reported feelings of sadness in terms of the previously introduced topical agenda of change (line 607). After another gap, the turn initial ('well') is coupled with an epistemic disclaimer, which again works to alert that there 'may be a problem with *how* the speaker is going to continue the second pair part turn and the recipient must figure out what the problem is in the course of the turn's unfolding' (Mazeland, 2016: 387). The interviewer produces a continuer and leaves a gap in which the child might add anything to his previous answer. When such a response is not forthcoming, the interviewer continues to produce a closing 'okay' that precedes the transition to the next question.

We have presented 3 fragments in this section that show how the children actively and repeatedly counter the suggestion that they have changed as a result of what happened. They may overtly disagree and emphasise a state of 'being essentially unchanged' (Fragment 3), disconfirm the scope of some changes and their relationship with what happened, and disagree with further questions that seek for personal changes (Fragment 4). Lastly, they may also present behaviour as previously existing, irrespective of what happened (Fragment 5) or by producing a 'mild' retraction, when prompted again to indicate a more precise area of change, by means of a claim to no knowledge.

How children resist the topical agenda that seeks to explore fundamental changes to the self, while also presenting claims of 'doing being recovered', is examined in the next section.

Presenting Normatively Preferred Versions of 'Doing Being Recovered'

In this section, we present two fragments in which the interviewing psychologist does not so much topicalise change in the question, but asks a more generally worded question. In Fragment 6 below, taken from the girl who was raped by a young boy from her town (see also Fragment 2), the interviewer has just inquired which advice the child would provide to other children who might have experienced a similar traumatic event (data not shown here: see also Lamerichs et al., 2015). After a continuer and a brief pause, the interviewer asks an 'and'-prefaced follow-up question that inquires what the girl would tell about herself to a peer (line 466). We will focus on how the ensuing self-description is constructed and how it attends to aspects of regained 'normality'.

Fragment 6

k20 - 'and that I also just tried...'

```
464  I:   hmhm;
          hmhm;
465       (1.5)
466  I:   en wat zou je hem vertellen over je z↑elf dan?
          and what would you tell him about yourself then?
467  K:   nou↓dat ik het ook >zelf m ee had gemaakt;<
          well that I had also >experienced it myself<;
468  K:   >dat ik ook gewoon< •h vervelende dingen had meegemaakt.
          >that I had also just< •h experienced unpleasant things.
469  K:   .h en dat ik ook gewoon heb geprobeerd om het steeds weer
          .h and that I also just tried again and again to
470  K:   .h >een beetje beter te maken<;
          .h >make it a little better<;
471  K:   >dat het steeds weer beter ging.<
          >that it improved bit by bit<.
472  K:   .h en dat ik uiteindelijk ook gewoon weer (.)
          .h and that eventually I am also just (.)
473  K:   .h gew↓oon kan doen.
          .h able to do normal things again.
474  I:   ja.
          yes.
475  K:   gewoon weer naar ((naam stad));
          just going to ((name town));
476  K:   langs het bos;
          walking along the woods;
477  K:   en- zonder lampje op mijn kamer,
          and- without the bedside lamp in my room,
478  I:   ja,
          yes,
479       (3.0)
480  I:   °hm°
          °hm°
481       (1.0)
482  I:   oke;
          okay;
```

In response to this question, the child orients first to the fact that she also experienced 'it', which is then rephrased more matter-of-factly as also 'just' having experienced 'unpleasant things' (line 468). Note how both lexical choices ('it', 'unpleasant things') leave ambiguous whether the child would specifically mention the nature of what happened to her peer, which might suggest its delicate nature (here, and in similar ways in other instances in this interview; cf. Silverman & Peräkylä, 1990). In lines 469–470, the girl stresses her attempts at improvement as a continuous and steady effort on her behalf to strive for the better. After attending to how her efforts turned into actual improvements (line 471), she stresses her current situation: it is presented as the ultimate goal of having reached an unproblematic state of 'regained normality' ('that eventually I am also just able to do normal things again', lines 472–473); or as being 'just the way she was'. What follows is a listed illustration that works as a set of evidential descriptions of 'resumed' activities that suggest a return to the normal and 'doing being ordinary' (lines 475–477). The interviewer produces an agreement token, and after a gap in which the child produces nothing further engages in closing work (line 482).

In Fragment 7 below, the interviewer has just asked the girl who was sexually assaulted (see also Fragment 1) whether her view of the world has changed, which the girl has disconfirmed (data not shown). The child is then invited to elaborate on a part of her answer. In lines 350–351, she formulates the gist of her answer in a minimal fashion ('pay a little more attention to it') and after a transition marker ('well', line 352) stresses its overall impact as non-consequential ('other than that it doesn't matter').

Fragment 7

k22 - 'I have to really stay alert'

```
350  K:  dus (.) daardoor ga je toch n- iets meer der op letten.
         so (.) because of that you do s- pay a little more attention to
it.
351      (.)
352  K:  nou (.) en >verder maakt het nie uit<.
         well (.) and >other than that it doesn't matter<.
353  I:  hmhm.
         hmhm.
354  I:  .hh en hoe let je der op;
         .hh and how do you pay attention to it;
355  K:  nou gewoon: (.) m- om te kijken,
         well just (.) m- to watch out,
356  K:  ik moet wel heel goed oppassen;
         I have to really stay alert;
357  K:  en niet iedereen zomaar gelo:ven,
         and not belief everybody just like that,
358  K:  want-=
         because-=
359  I:  =hmhm
         =hmhm
360  K:  .h (1.0) mensen die je goed kent;
         .h (1.0) people you know well;
361  K:  die kun je wel geloven,
         you can believe them,
362  K:  alleen mensen die je niet goed ke:nt,
         only people you don't know well,
363  K:  die moet je echt niet geloven;
         you should really not believe them;
364  K:  moet je eerst ↑vra:gen,
         you should ask first,
365  I:  ja;
         yes;
366      (3)
367  I:  °oke.°
         °okay.°
```

After a continuer, the interviewer asks a more generally worded follow-up question that related to the topic raised by the child ('and how do you pay attention to it', line 354), which demonstrates that she might not be sufficiently satisfied with the answer given. The follow-up question seeks an explicit elaboration of exactly how the child engages in her current behaviour. The child's response is prefaced with 'well' and 'just' (line 355) which marks the answer as not straightforward and possibly also hearable as a slight critique of the self-evident nature of the interviewer's question (Schegloff & Lerner, 2009). She continues by answering the how question with an account (as if it was a 'why' question), offering an explanation couched in verbs of necessity (lines 356–357) as well as constructing it as a generic explanation ('you should really not believe them; you should ask first', lines 360–364). The verbs of necessity ('must') and emphasis ('only', 'really', lines 362–363) construct her response as a set of normatively preferred lessons or directives (cf. Keevallik, 2011). The normativity not only suggests that the child has actively sought ways to prevent what happened from happening again but also attend to her current situation as 'doing being recovered'.

In this final section, it was demonstrated that children, when asked to elaborate on their current situation (Fragment 6), account for their behaviour in terms that are normatively preferred (Fragment 7). When asked how they would describe themselves to a peer, they present converting to the normal ('how things were before it happened') in a way that demonstrates recovery as something they were able to achieve.

Concluding Remarks

This chapter has shown that eliciting children's perspectives on how they have experienced a traumatic occurrence and inviting them to do so *in their own words* may be met with some unforeseen challenges. Although the interviewing psychologist, faced with the difficult task of asking about sensitive issues, may want to provide some necessary leeway or guidance to the child for answering (i.e. introducing the experiences of other children in the question preface as something to 'latch on to' in the response), the children in our data show conversational strategies of resisting the topical agenda and the presuppositions that underpin the psychologist's questions.

A close examination of our data enabled us to detail three sets of interrelated practices children engage in, when responding to the questions of the interviewing psychologist: they may present downgraded descriptions of what happened to them, they may discount assumptions that they have changed in a fundamental way as a result of the traumatic experience, and they may volunteer normatively preferred accounts of change to demonstrate 'doing being recovered'.

We examined these practices in three sections. In section "Presenting Downgraded Versions of What Happened", we showed how children, while able to provide detailed descriptions of what happened, subtly countered ascriptions of being different or strange. When responding to questions that inquire whether there are positive lessons to be drawn from what happened, children resist this topical agenda and offer a downplayed account that presents what happened as merely coincidental. The traumatic occurrence is thus constructed as belonging to the category of events that do not have the imprint that allow for such lessons to be learned. Secondly, in section "Discounting Ascriptions of a Changed Self" we demonstrated how children clearly recount the suggestion that the traumatic occurrence has caused them to change in any meaningful way. Interestingly, they continue these discounting practices even when the question of change is put to them on multiple occasions and formatted in ways that clearly seek a confirming response. It was shown how children may agree to minor changes in behaviour, retract their initial answers to demonstrate the absence of a more fundamental type of change, as well as emphasise 'sameness' and an essentially unchanged self. Lastly, section "Presenting Normatively Preferred Versions of 'Doing Being Recovered'" examined how children volunteer descriptive accounts of change, and when they do so they attend to offering normatively preferred, agentic scenarios of recovery which equal 'doing being recovered'. These scenarios worked to emphasise 'regained normality' and 'doing being recovered' as the current state of being. Taken together, these strategies show how children perform identity work around the notion of 'a changed self', which seems contingent upon whether account of change is volunteered (Fragment 6) or explicitly asked for.

Overall, this chapter has demonstrated the strategies children employ to subtly criticise and resist the trajectory of particular questions (most notably questions that inquire after personal change) as well as the presuppositional basis of other questions (i.e. constructing the children as 'odd' or different because of what happened, or the traumatic occurrence as an important occasion for learning lessons). The 'layered' structure of many of the questions that were asked in these interviews (i.e. formatted as prefaced questions or alternative questions and coupled by polar questions or how questions) seems to even increase their presuppositional basis. Rather than functioning as a helping, 'neutral' device that facilitates the broadest possible repertoire of answers from the child, these 'layered' questions are also often met with strategies of resistance. Hence, the setting of the psychological research interview, emphasising question formats that put special weight on 'change' and 'recovery', run the risk of 'offering up its own agendas and categories and getting those same agendas and categories back in a refined or filtered or inverted form' (Potter & Hepburn, 2005: 291). More importantly, when attempting to elicit the unique perspective of the child, these psychological interviews seem to offer little room to appreciate more fully the interactional concerns of the child, which we have shown to be clearly oriented to identity work and the moral implications that are embedded in the interviewer's question formats.

Professional Reflection

Eva Alisic

Abstract

Although child traumatic stress is increasingly recognised as a public health concern, the perspectives of children who have been affected are still underrepresented and underutilised. A common example of impeding adult concerns is the belief that talking about trauma with children is 're-traumatising' them, even though this has been debunked in research.

The current reflection considers two main lessons learned from interviews with children who experienced trauma. First, children demonstrate agency through their nuanced and detailed accounts of experiences, including effective negations of suggestions by the interviewer. Second, while interviews are characterised by a lack of information (e.g. about our conversation partner and their expectations) and substantial cognitive load (e.g. formulating questions while listening and keeping track of interview objectives), there are enticing opportunities for testing and improving question formulation. Ongoing development in this domain can help ensure that children's voices are really understood, heard and acted upon.

Exposure to potentially traumatic events is unfortunately common among children and adolescents. By their 18th birthday, the majority of young people have been confronted with the loss of a loved one, a car crash, an assault or another type of trauma (Copeland, Keeler, Angold, & Costello, 2007). Although child traumatic stress is more and more often recognised as a major public health concern, the perspectives of children who have been affected are still underrepresented and underutilised. In a few areas, concerns about this lack of attention to children's views have been expressed explicitly. For example, Callaghan and colleagues work with children exposed to domestic violence and write that 'the failure to talk to children and young people about their lived experiences of domestic violence underestimates their capacity for agency' (2017: 3371). Moreover, they reiterate that 'adult concerns about young people's vulnerabilities and inability to safely reflect on their experiences can lead to institutionally imposed gatekeeping, resulting in silencing or tokenistic participation'.

A common example of impeding adult concerns is the widely held belief that talking about trauma with children is 're-traumatising' them, even though this has been debunked in research (see, e.g., Kassam-Adams & Newman, 2005). Of course, conversations about trauma need to be respectful (e.g. giving the interviewee time to settle into the interview; asking questions that are needed, not because they provide 'juicy' details that do not serve a purpose), and with referral options in case needs are identified, but in themselves they are not re-traumatising. The risk of not asking children about their perspectives is that prevention and intervention efforts cannot be optimally adapted to children's needs. In contrast to prevailing adult concerns, children have a capacity for agency, which they showed in the current chapter as well.

Children's Agency

The chapter contains two main lessons or insights for me. First, as mentioned, that children have and demonstrate agency. They showed that they were able to provide nuanced and detailed accounts of experiences. They also showed that they could effectively disagree or negate suggestions made by the interviewer (me). This is incredibly promising information, since this means that with careful listening and analysing of both the interview content and the interactional context, we will be able to harvest and better understand children's views. It also means that we are getting different responses and novel information compared to just going with what we think of something as adults. Children truly bring their own unique perspective. In other words, their contributions lead to different information compared to if we just 'made it up' as adults. This is important and reinforces the point above that we should support children in having a voice.

However, as Lundy (2007) indicates, having a voice in itself is not enough. In line with a children's rights perspective, children also need a genuine audience, space and influence. For us as researchers and practitioners, this means that there is a responsibility to ensure that children's perspectives reach further than just our own professional publications. In the case of the interviews included in this chapter, we have integrated children's perspectives in a toolkit for primary school teachers and in a book for both parents and professionals on supporting children after trauma. Some of the interviews we have taken further, to education opportunities and to policy makers. There is still ample room to do more in this respect.

Improvements in Question Formulation

In terms of the second lesson, the chapter emphasises and highlights that there is still substantial scope for improvement in question formulation. It shows, in line with other CA research, that interviews can be analysed in a detailed manner, leading to fascinating insights in interview dynamics. While this work would be incredibly useful in my field of psychotraumatology, it is considered relatively infrequently, even though there are some very practical implications flowing from the analyses. An example in this chapter is the prefaced question with regard to the child experiencing positive aspects (or any potential experience, really). The question raised an expectation for an answer confirming experiencing something positive. It would be relatively easy to expand that question to also include the mention of children who did *not* experience change. Presenting both options before asking how it is for the child might give the child a much more 'neutral' starting position for their answer.

As the actual interviewer, I have some insight into the thoughts that went through my head during the interviews, something that is consciously not part of the analysis presented. My personal memory—as biased as it maybe—is that I did not necessarily mean to emphasise that children can experience positive change. Rather, I came from a slight feeling of awkwardness about asking a child who had clearly gone through a horrible experience, about positive consequences. By mentioning that some children had experienced positive things, I somehow aimed to defend myself from the potential criticism of asking such a naïve question that anything good could have come from that experience.

Dancing in the Dark During Interviews

As interview partners, we are all still 'dancing in the dark' in these conversations. My intentions were not clear from my words, children might have interpreted my words in ways that differ from what I expected, and in the analyses, we interpret children's reactions in ways that may not be in line with their original intentions. While we—the child and I—are conducting the interview, this means that we are working (dancing) with limited information, about our conversation partner and about relevant circumstances outside of the interview. The same applies to limited information about each other's expectations of the interview. For example, children have ideas about what the interviewer wants to hear. I sometimes suspected that children in our interviews felt they had to 'perform' and show that they had well understood the therapy they had received. Some thoughts that the children expressed (e.g. 'it could have happened to someone else', line 743, indicating that it was not personally targeted, that she was not to blame) might have been informed by therapy and repeated, to consciously or unconsciously live up to the presumed expectations of the interviewer (of note, some of the children had received therapy in the psychotrauma centre where the interviews took place, possibly even reinforcing this tendency).

Also, my impression is that things happen so quickly in an interview that children nor adults are fully aware or in charge of what they are doing. For example, as an interviewer, there is substantial cognitive load to do with thinking ahead, thinking back to what has already been said, formulating a question in the best possible way under the circumstances, listening in the moment, while linking answers to each other, thinking about potential gaps that need to be further explored, and checking whether everything is on track. The effects of this load can be multiple; they might affect the quality of listening, and therefore the response to information that children volunteered. They might also affect the formulation of questions: sometimes, I found myself thinking aloud in order to formulate a question. In itself, thinking aloud is sometimes taught as a technique in clinical psychology (it can have various useful functions in relationship building) and I sometimes employ it for that reason. However, my guess is that a part of it was also still working through the best way to word a question, despite the fact that my co-researchers and I had conducted mock interviews beforehand and held ongoing feedback sessions during the study. It may be of interest to conduct further analyses to assess how the formulation of questions evolves over a series of interviews with the same topic list. My expectation would be that questions become more 'fluent', and hopefully open, over time.

'Good Questions'

Is a question only 'good' if a child agrees with it? Is a question by definition 'wrong' if a child disagrees? The fact that a child feels comfortable enough to say no is possibly also a positive sign. This may not be the case in all interviews or conversations. Maybe exploring the boundaries of what a child agrees with involves seeking negative answers. In interviews such as in the current chapter, in which one is really interested in children's perspective, I can imagine that one can develop a specific protocol for the start of the interview that reinforces the child's capacity to disagree. For example, one or more questions can be designed to a lead to a disagreement by the child (e.g. asking a question about their clothes, referring to the wrong colour), followed by praise for the courage to disagree and a reinforcement that disagreement in the remainder of the interview is absolutely fine. Such a protocol could be tested and refined in research settings.

More generally, the types of question formulations discussed in the current chapter seem to lend themselves well to a more experimental set-up, while not detracting from the value of the interviews in themselves. With more training and careful development, we could pre-formulate, for example, 3 different questions in 3 different ways and test these versions over a range of interviews. With the original set of interviews drawn from for the current chapter, we could have texted each of the formulations in 8 children. It would remain a semi-structured interview, but it would have a small number of set questions within it. This would allow to better understand the differences in interactions following the question formulation within the context of trauma recovery narratives.

Finally, a developmental lens seems of value in the context of (improving) the interviews. Would the same questions work with a 5-year old, and with a 15-year old? In our case, the interviews were with children aged 8–12 years old; in the first few years of primary school. Understanding of questions, and vocabulary to answer them and address complex emotional issues develop over time (see, e.g., Salmon & Bryant, 2002), and are likely to lead to different interview dynamics. Thinking of the prefaced design that was central in the current analyses, an even lengthier version as I proposed above, is likely to be difficult to follow for a younger child. Considering the importance of understanding children's perspectives, it is crucial that we better understand the dynamics, intricacies and boundaries of conversations such as clinical and research interviews, and adapt our practices over time to ensure that children's voices are really understood, heard and acted upon.

References

Alisic, E., Boeije, H. R., Jongmans, M. J., & Kleber, R. J. (2011). Children's perspectives on dealing with traumatic events. *Journal of Loss and Trauma: International Perspectives on Stress & Coping, 16*(6), 477–496.

American Psychiatric Association. (2000). *Diagnostic and statistical manual of mental disorders IV—Text revision.* Washington, DC: American Psychiatric Association.

Beach, W. (1993). Transitional regularities for 'casual' "okay" usages. *Journal of Pragmatics, 19*(4), 325–352.

Bergmann, J. R. (1998). Introduction: Morality in discourse. *Research on Language and Social Interaction, 31*(3–4), 279–294.

Blakely, H., & Moles, K. (2016). Interviewing in the 'interview society': Making visible the biographical work of producing accounts for interviews. *Qualitative Research, 17*(2), 159–172.

Boyd, E., & Heritage, J. (2006). Taking the history: Questioning during comprehensive history taking. In J. Heritage & D. Maynard (Eds.), *Communication in medical care: Interactions between primary care physicians and patients* (pp. 151–184). Cambridge, UK: Cambridge University Press.

Buttny, R. (2003). *Social accountability in communication.* London, UK: Sage.

Callaghan, J. E. M., Fellin, L. C., Mavrou, S., Alexander, J., & Sixsmith, J. (2017). The management of disclosure in children's accounts of domestic violence: Practices of telling and not telling. *Journal of Child and Family Studies, 26*(12), 3370–3387.

Childs, C., & Walsh, D. (2017). Self-disclosure and self-deprecating self-reference: Conversational practices of personalization in police interviews with children reporting alleged sexual offences. *Journal of Pragmatics, 121,* 188–201.

Clark, J., & Richards, S. (2017). The cherished conceits of research with children: Does seeking the agentic voice of the child through participatory methods deliver what it promises? *Sociological Studies of Children and Youth, 22*(1), 127–147.

Clift, R. (2001). Meaning in interaction: the Case of actually. *Language, 77*(2), 245–291. www.jstor.org/stable/3086775.

Copeland, W. E., Keeler, G., Angold, A., & Costello, E. J. (2007). Traumatic events and posttraumatic stress in childhood. *Archives of General Psychiatry, 64*(5), 577–584.

Cromdal, J., Danby, S., Emmison, M., Osvaldsson, K., & Cobb-Moore. (2017). "Basically it's the usual whole teen girl thing": Stage-of-life categories on a children and young people's helpline. *Symbolic Interaction, 41*(1), 25–44.
Danby, S., & Baker, C. (1998). "What's the problem?" Restoring social order in the preschool classroom. In I. Hutchby & J. Moran-Ellis (Eds.), *Children and social competence: Arenas of action* (pp. 157–186). London, UK: Falmer Press.
Freed, A., & Ehrlich, S. (Eds.). (2010). *Why do you ask?: The function of questions in institutional discourse.* Oxford, UK: Oxford University Press.
Halkowski, T. (1998). Patients smoking counts: Implications of quantification practices. *Journal of General Internal Medicine, 13*(1), 107.
Halkowski, T. (2006). Realizing the illness: Patients' narratives of symptom discovery. In P. Drew, M. Harness-Goodwin, J. Gumperz, & D. Schiffrin (Series Eds.) and J. Heritage & D. Maynard (Vol. Eds.), *Communication in medical care: Interactions between primary care physicians and patients.* Studies in Interactional Sociolinguistics (Vol. 20, pp. 86–114). Cambridge, UK: Cambridge University Press.
Hepburn, A., & Bolden, G. (2013). The conversation analytic approach to transcription. In J. Sidnell & T. Stivers (Eds.), *The handbook of conversation analysis* (pp. 57–76). Oxford, UK: Wiley-Blackwell.
Heritage, J. (2002). The limits of questioning: Negative interrogatives and hostile question content. *Pragmatics, 34*(10–11), 1427–1446.
Heritage, J. (2010). Questioning in Medicine. In A. Freed & S. Ehrlich (Eds.), *Why do you ask?: The function of questions in institutional discourse* (pp. 42–68). Oxford, UK: Oxford University Press.
Hutchby, I. (2005). Children's talk and social competence. *Children and Society, 19*(1), 66–73.
Hutchby, I. (2007). *The discourse of child counselling: Impact studies in Language and Society.* Amsterdam: John Benjamins Publishing Company.
Hutchby, I. (2015). Therapeutic vision: Eliciting talk about feelings in child counselling for family separation. In M. O'Reilly & J. N. Lester (Eds.), *The Palgrave Handbook of Child Mental Health: Discourse and Conversation Studies* (pp. 541–558). Basingstoke, UK: Palgrave Macmillan.
Hutchby, I., & O'Reilly, M. (2010). Children's participation and the familial moral order in family therapy. *Discourse Studies, 12*(1), 49–64.
Hutchby, I., & Wooffitt, R. (2008). *Conversation analysis* (2nd ed.). Oxford, UK: Blackwell.
Iversen, C. (2014). 'I don't know if I should believe him': Knowledge and believability in interviews with children. *British Journal of Social Psychology, 53*(2), 367–386.

Jefferson, G. (2004). "At first I thought": A normalizing device for extraordinary events. In G. Lerner (Eds.), *Conversation analysis: Studies from the first generation* (pp. 131–167). Amsterdam: Benjamins.

Kassam-Adams, N., & Newman, E. (2005). Child and parent reactions to participation in clinical research. *General Hospital Psychiatry, 27*(1), 29–35.

Keevallik, L. (2011). The terms of not knowing. In T. Stivers, L. Mondada, & J. Steensig (Eds.), *The morality of knowledge in conversation* (pp. 184–206). Cambridge, UK: Cambridge University Press.

Kidwell, M. (2009). What happened?: An epistemics of before and after in "at-the-scene" police questioning. *Research on Language and Social Interaction, 42*(1), 20–41.

Lamerichs, J. Alisic, E., & Schasfoort, M. (2015). 'You just have to be cheerful really': Children's accounts of ordinariness in trauma recovery talk. In M. O'Reilly & J. N. Lester (Eds.), *The Palgrave handbook of child mental health: Discourse and conversation studies* (pp. 618–635). Basingstoke, UK: Palgrave Macmillan.

Lamerichs, J., Alisic, E., & Schasfoort, M. (2018). Accounts and their epistemic implications: How children's 'I don't know' answers are received in trauma recovery talk. *Research on Children and Social Interaction, 2*(1), 25–48.

Lester, J. N. (2014). Negotiating abnormality/normality in therapy talk: A discursive psychology approach to the study of therapeutic interactions and children with autism. *Qualitative Psychology, 1*(2), 178–193.

Lundy, L. (2007). 'Voice'is not enough: Conceptualising Article 12 of the United Nations Convention on the Rights of the Child. *British Educational Research Journal, 33*(6), 927–942.

Mazeland, H. (2003). *Inleididng in de conversatie-analyse* [Introduction to conversation analysis]. Bussum, The Netherlands: Coutinho.

Mazeland, H. (2016). The positionally sensitive workings of the Dutch particle 'nou'. In P. Auer & Y. Maschler (Eds.), *Nu/Nä: A family of discourse markers across the language of Europe and beyond* (pp. 377–408). Berlin and Boston: Walter de Gruyter.

Noordegraaf, M., Van Nijnatten, C., & Elbers, E. (2009). Assessing candidates for adoptive parenthood: Institutional re-formulations of biographical notes. *Children and Youth Services Review, 31*(1), 89–96.

O'Reilly, M., & Lester, J. (2015). *The Palgrave handbook of child mental health.* London, UK: Palgrave Macmillan.

Pomerantz, A. (1984). Agreeing and disagreeing with assessments: Some features of preferred/dispreferred turn shapes. In J. M. Atkinson & J. Heritage (Eds.),

Structures of social action (pp. 57–101). Cambridge: Cambridge University Press.

Potter, J., & Hepburn, A. (2005). Qualitative interviews in psychology: Problems and possibilities. *Qualitative Research in Psychology, 2*(4), 281–307.

Sacks, H. (1984). On doing "being ordinary". In J. M. Atkinson & J. Heritage (Eds.), *Structures of social action: Studies in conversation analysis* (pp. 413–429). Cambridge, UK: Cambridge University Press.

Salmon, K., & Bryant, R. A. (2002). Posttraumatic stress disorder in children: The influence of developmental factors. *Clinical Psychological Review, 22*(2), 163–188.

Schegloff, E., & Lerner, G. (2009). Beginning to respond: Well-prefaced responses to wh-questions. *Research on Language and Social Interaction, 42*(2), 91–115.

Silverman, D. (2017). How was it for you? The Interview Society and the irresistible rise of the (poorly analysed) interview. *Qualitative Research, 17*(2), 144–158.

Silverman, D., & Peräkylä, A. (1990). AIDS-counselling: The interactional organization of talk about 'delicate' issues. *Sociology of Health and Illness, 12*(3), 293–318.

Stafford, V., Hutchby, I., Karim, I., & O'Reilly, M. (2016). "Why are you here?" Seeking children's accounts of their presentation to Child and Adolescent Mental Health Service (CAMHS). *Clinical Child Psychology and Psychiatry, 2*(1), 3–18.

Terr, L. (1990). *Too scared to cry*. New York: Harper and Row.

Urman, M. L., Funk, J. B., & Elliot, R. (2001). Children's experiences of traumatic events: The negotiation of normalcy and difference. *Clinical Child Psychology and Psychiatry, 6*(3), 403–424.

van Nijnatten, C. (2013). Downgrading as a counterstrategy: A case study in child welfare. *Child and Family Social Work, 18*(2), 139–148.

Van Wesel, F., Boeije, H., Alisic, E., & Drost, S. (2012). I'll be working my way back: A qualitative synthesis on the trauma experience of children. *Psychological Trauma: Research, Practice and Policy, 4*(5), 516–526.

8

Children and Mental Health Talk: Perspectives on Social Competence—An Epilogue

Karin Osvaldsson Cromdal and Jakob Cromdal

At first glance, "mental health talk" may have an adult ring to it, as indeed does the notion of "children's social competence". Evidently, both concepts are adult constructs and may have little to do with what children themselves orient to in the course of everyday life. The question then arises whether a book thus titled can tell us anything at all about the social worlds of children who are parties to talk that concerns their mental health and well-being. The plain answer is yes, but one will need to read beyond the title.

In fact, all the chapters offer insight into how children handle themselves in interactional encounters with adults, and occasionally also with other children (cf. Theobald & Danby), where focus is on various aspects

K. Osvaldsson Cromdal (✉) · J. Cromdal
Department of Social and Welfare Studies (ISV), Linköping University, Norrköping, Sweden
e-mail: karin.osvaldsson@liu.se

J. Cromdal
e-mail: jakob.cromdal@liu.se

J. Lamerichs et al. (eds.), *Children and Mental Health Talk*, The Language of Mental Health,
https://doi.org/10.1007/978-3-030-28426-8_8

of the children's mental health and well-being. What is more, this insight is a product of rigorous analysis of interaction informed by the sibling scholarly traditions of ethnomethodology and conversation analysis EM/CA. This typically means that the insight on offer is highly praxeological (Mondada, 2011) that is, soundly anchored in close empirical observation of participants' own practices rather than generated by research hypotheses or coding schemes infused with, say, theories of child development. In this respect, the authors all align with Sacks' dictum to use "observation as a basis for theorizing" (1971/1992: 420).

However, careful commitment to key aspects of interactional organisation is not news—it is a long-standing trademark of EM/CA inquiry. Much less commonplace is what we learn from the book about mental health talk. It broadens the concept considerably, by showing that dealing with issues of mental health and well-being is sometimes the job of professionals who are not necessarily qualified in a mental health profession. To a large extent, this is due to EM/CA's rejection of a "container" view of context (also known as "bucket" theory of context, e.g. Goodwin & Heritage, 1990), according to which a certain type of institutional talk would be determined by the institutional setting in which it takes place. Instead, EM/CA scholars point to the reflexive relationship between the setting and the actions that take place there. As the chapters of this book demonstrate, mental health talk with children does indeed take place in different clinical (Kawashima & Maynard; O'Reilly, Kiyimba & Hutchby) and clinically oriented research settings (Lamerichs, Alisic & Schasfoort), just as it takes place in other institutional contexts such as police interrogations (Jol, Stommel & Spooren), video-solicited research interviews with school children (Theobald & Danby), or during urban excursions in preschool groups (Bateman & Danby).

But what about children's social competence? A brief historical overview may help to situate the contribution of the book's chapters. It is thirty years since James and Prout's (1990) introduction of the "New social studies of childhood" (NSSC), a research programme that has had a strong impact on sociological understandings of childhood and proved consequential in establishing what is known as the "competence paradigm" (Hutchby & Moran Ellis, 1998) in contemporary child studies. NSSC offered a long-overdue reaction to the default developmental orientation to children's competence, as well as a prevailing conceptualisation of childhood as above all a period of socialisation, whereby adults secure the child's transformation from an "incipient being" (Durkheim, 1911) to a full member of society. It is worth noting that there had been earlier attempts in ethnomethodology (e.g. Mackay, 1974; Sacks, 1966/1992; Speier, 1970, 1976) to instate the child as an active agent in sociological work, by pointing to the adult bias hosted within socialisation theories. For instance, in an essay on adult-child interaction, which he described in terms of culture contact, Speier argued that

> the classical formulation of socialisation [...] is an interpretive imposition of adult lay conceptions onto the data of childhood behaviours, taking, as it were, only half of the interactional picture into consideration. The children's half, that part of the interactional picture not represented by the ideology, has been left unformulated in the analysis. (1976: 99)

In a similar vein, Mackay (1974) proposed that

> [children's] competence is not acknowledged within the normative approach because the study of socialisation takes the views of the dominant culture (adult) and proposes them as scientific findings. (p. 180)

This dominant adult culture is rooted in lay understandings of children—understandings that, according to Garfinkel, Girton, Livingston, and Sacks (1962/1982), were heavily infused with a developmental stance to the conduct of children

> Within that relationship [adults vs. children], which entails the adults' use of the developmental scheme as a part, children are naturally, normally, obviously, objectively, really and observably faulted speakers. Further, their faulted speech is observably the present phase of a projected and familiar course. They speak as they do, being on their way to speaking one day better than they currently do: one day they will speak like the adults. (p. 4)

In essence, this developmental "scheme" provides for a view of children as "adults-in-becoming" (Garfinkel et al., 1962/1982: 2). As a product of socialisation theory and an almost mandatory developmental perspective, the adult bias in studies of children effectively denied the possibility of seeing their competence (see Cromdal, 2009, for a more recent sample). As it turned out, this critique of the state of affairs in social and behavioural studies of children was far before its time and did not gain much foothold outside ethnomethodology. Yet, decades later, the very same arguments echoed in James and Prout's prescription list for a new generation of social studies of childhood:

> 3. Children's social relationships and cultures are worthy of study in their own right, independent of the perspective and concerns of adults.
>
> 4. Children are and must be seen as active in the construction and determination of their own social lives, the lives of those around them and of the societies in which they live. (Prout & James, 1990: 8)

There is, of course, a danger in *a priori* ascriptions of competence of tipping the scales the other way, but at the very least the programmatic claims of NSSC sparked a sound discussion concerning the view of children in both sociology and psychology. In childhood psychology (Sommer, 2012) for instance, the universally acknowledged developmental theories are now being challenged and the psychological life of children and young persons is understood in its cultural and social context, rather than mapped onto an idealised developmental trajectory towards adulthood. Consequently, the image of the child as inherently fragile and lacking in various abilities is abandoned, without being replaced by an ideology of competence. Instead, the concept of the resilience is proposed, where childhood and children's individual experiences are always set in relation to the surrounding context (Sommer, 2012).

Two of the chapters in this volume examine aspects of social competence in the course of clinical assessment. Kawashima and Maynard focus on the local organisation of echolalia—a form of repetition, traditionally seen as an indicator of communicative impairment—showing how its delivery resulted in a tweaking and expanding of the standardised testing sequences, allowing the child to produce relevant tasks and "adjust to the requirements of the institutional setting" (p. 70). The chapter by O'Reilly,

Kiyimba and Hutchby, focuses on young clients' problem presentations in mental health assessments. The client's competence was initially presumed, and recognised, when the accounts of trouble were grounded in the client's own emotions and experiences—their personal epistemic domain. However, when the accounts intersected with the clinical epistemic domain, for instance if clients used a diagnostic term to describe their problems, clinicians would inquire the details of that account. At the crossroads of personal and professional knowledge then, young clients were simultaneously credited with social competence as well as held accountable for aspiring to use medical terminology.

In the research interviews examined by Lamerichs, Alisic and Schasfoort, the interviewing psychologist, who was trying to elicit the children's perspectives on traumatic events in the past, faced an interactional challenge: the respondents were reluctant to align with the presuppositions hosted in the interviewer's questions. The children's social competence that emerges from the analysis is not about their ability to describe and reflect on their problems but in the various techniques they deployed to control the conversational topics and to construct a narrative in which the psychological consequences of the traumatic event were downplayed (cf. Evans and Maines, 1995). Narrative competence is also in focus in the police interviews with child witnesses of sexual abuse examined by Jol, Stommel and Spooren. Here, we learn how children report having tricked the alleged sex offender in various ways that demonstrate high degree of creativity, social competence and situational awareness. In the context of sexual abuse and violence, there is a common belief—known as the ultimate resistance myth (Estrich, 1987)—that true victims always put up extreme resistance. According to the authors, by presenting the police officers with narrative accounts that highlight their agency and the rationality of misleading the alleged offender, the children orient themselves to this expectation and pre-empt the possibility of being blamed for not having resisted more forcefully.

When a natural disaster hits a community, adults and children alike are affected. The chapter by Bateman and Danby examines how teachers and children at a preschool in Christchurch (New Zealand) engage in working through the experience in the aftermath of the recent earthquakes, while walking around in the city. The analysis shows how the material environment is brought about in situ to make space for even the smallest of children's reflections about the devastating consequences of the catastrophe. In the chapter by Theobald and Danby, the setting is a research group interview with preschool children where the researcher has asked the participating children to reflect upon an earlier video recording of a play situation. While watching the video, the children produced different opinions about what really happened and how the participants had really felt during the play. With the other chapters in mind, this analysis takes a somewhat different tack on mental health talk, showing how the researcher seeks to steer the interaction away from reflecting upon the play events, to handling the emerging situation so that a traumatising experience of the interview is avoided.

Although the notion of children's social competence is being iterated throughout this book, it is important, as some of the professional commentaries remind us, to bear in mind that mental health talk is an engagement of at least two parties, both bringing to the event their traits, experiences and competencies, as well as presuppositions concerning the competencies of the other (cf. Waksler, 1986). As we learn from several studies in this book, the professionals skillfully work to enhance children's participation in the interaction by exploiting the conversational machinery described by Sacks, Schegloff, and Jefferson (1974), to project and make conditionally relevant certain courses of actions in the subsequent turns at talk. The studies in this book thus avoid focusing single-mindedly on the one side, recognising it a shaky ground on which to build an understanding of any professional practice.

Crucially, the EM/CA approach adopted in the analyses may safeguard against overembracing the "competence paradigm" concerning the status of children as well as offer important theoretical leverage to a sociological understanding of institutional practice. Its approach to social interaction is participant-oriented and, at the same time, free from analytically intuitive lifespan categories. Preschoolers, adolescents, 40-somethings or gold agers alike are treated in the first place as participants to interaction, relieving the analysis of the—often unreflected—burden of premature categorisation. This does not suggest that analysts are ignorant of the possible relevance of cognitive functioning—and whatever competence, power, experience and what not, that may be conventionally associated with it—only that such status is analytically treated as an issue of membership categorisation, that is, a strictly interactional achievement.

What is at stake here for those taking a scholarly or professional interest in work with children's mental health and well-being is the relevance and status of child-ness and adult-ness, of lay-ness and professional-ness, of social competence and empathy in the situated conduct that constitutes this work. With its Schutzean heritage, EM/CA treats social reality as an issue of intersubjective relationships. Such relationships are products of "the reasoning structures and conventional member-orientations involved in […] empirically observed courses of social interaction" (Coulter, 1979: 20). Of course, the enterprise does not allow us to understand what it may feel like to be a child client or an adult professional in a diagnostic, therapeutic or counselling session focusing on one party's traumatic experience or some other aspect of mental health. What it does promise is to demonstrate how subjective matters are explicated and made sense of by other parties and how such sensemaking bears on the work being carried out. In the course of analysis, we often get to learn a thing or two about the institution in which that work takes place.

References

Coulter, J. (1979). *The social construction of mind: Studies in ethnomethodology and linguistic philosophy*. London: Macmillan.

Cromdal, J. (2009). Childhood and social interaction in everyday life—An introduction. *Journal of Pragmatics, 41*(8), 1473–1476.

Durkheim, E. (1911/1979). Childhood. In W. S. F. Pickering (Eds.), *Essays on morals and education*. London: Routledge & Kegan Paul.

Estrich, S. (1987). *Real rape*. Cambridge, MA: Harvard University Press.

Evans, W. J., & Maines, D. R. (1995). Narrative structures and the analysis of incest. *Symbolic Interaction, 18*(3), 303–322.

Garfinkel, H., Girton, G., Livingston, E., & Sacks, H. (1962/1982). *Studies of kids' culture and kids' talk* (Unpublished manuscript). University of California, Los Angeles.

Goodwin, C., & Heritage, J. (1990). Conversation analysis. *Annual Review of Anthropology, 19*(1), 283–307.

Hutchby, I., & Moran-Ellis, J. (Eds.). (1998). *Children and social competence: Arenas of action*. London: Falmer.
James, A., & Prout, A. (Eds.). (1990). *Constructing and reconstructing childhood: Contemporary issues in the sociological study of childhood*. London: Falmer.
Mackay, R. W. (1974). Conceptions of children and models of socialization. In R. Turner (Ed.), *Ethnomethodology*. Harmondsworth: Penguin.
Mondada, L. (2011). Understanding as an embodied, situated and sequential achievement in interaction. *Journal of Pragmatics, 43*(2), 542–552.
Prout, A., & James, A. (1990). A new paradigm for the Sociology of childhood? Provenance, promise and problems. In A. James & A. Prout (Eds.), *Constructing and reconstructing childhood: Contemporary issues in the sociological study of childhood*. London: Falmer.
Sacks, H. (1966/1992). *Lectures on conversation* (Vol. 1). Oxford: Blackwell.
Sacks, H. (1971/1992). *Lectures on conversation* (Vol. 2). Oxford: Blackwell.
Sacks, H., Schegloff, E. A., & Jefferson, G. (1974). A simplest systematics for the organization of turn taking for conversation. *Language, 50*(4), 696–735.
Sommer, D. (2012). *A childhood psychology: Young children in changing times*. Basingstoke: Palgrave Macmillan.
Speier, M. (1970). The everyday world of the child. In J. Douglas (Ed.), *Understanding everyday life*. Chicago: Aldine.
Speier, M. (1976). The child as conversationalist: Some culture contact features of conversational interactions between adults and children. In M. Hammersley & P. Woods (Eds.), *The process of schooling* (pp. 98–103). London: Routledge & Kegan Paul.
Waksler, F. C. (1986). Studying children: Phenomenological insights. *Human Studies, 9*(1), 71–82.

Index

J. Lamerichs et al. (eds.), *Children and Mental Health Talk*, The Language of Mental Health,
https://doi.org/10.1007/978-3-030-28426-8

FSC
www.fsc.org
MIX
Papier | Fördert gute Waldnutzung
FSC® C083411

Kolibri 360 GmbH
Ferdinand-Jühlke-Straße 7
99095 Erfurt, Deutschland
produktsicherheit@kolibri360.de